AF887590

It's easy to get lost in the cancer world

Let NCCN Guidelines for Patients® be your guide

- ✓ Step-by-step guides to the cancer care options likely to have the best results
- ✓ Based on treatment guidelines used by health care providers worldwide
- ✓ Designed to help you discuss cancer treatment with your doctors

About

National Comprehensive Cancer Network®

NCCN Guidelines for Patients® are developed by the National Comprehensive Cancer Network® (NCCN®)

NCCN®

- An alliance of 28 leading cancer centers across the United States devoted to patient care, research, and education

Cancer centers that are part of NCCN:
NCCN.org/cancercenters

NCCN Clinical Practice Guidelines in Oncology (NCCN Guidelines®)

- Developed by doctors from NCCN cancer centers using the latest research and years of experience
- For providers of cancer care all over the world
- Expert recommendations for cancer screening, diagnosis, and treatment

Free online at
NCCN.org/guidelines

NCCN Guidelines for Patients®

- Present information from the NCCN Guidelines in an easy-to-learn format
- For people with cancer and those who support them
- Explain the cancer care options likely to have the best results

NCCN Quick Guide™ Sheets

- Key points from the NCCN Guidelines for Patients

Free online at
NCCN.org/patientguidelines

NATIONAL COMPREHENSIVE CANCER NETWORK FOUNDATION
Guiding Treatment. Changing Lives.

and supported by funding from NCCN Foundation®

These guidelines are based on the NCCN Clinical Practice Guidelines in Oncology (NCCN Guidelines®) for Non-Small Cell Lung Cancer (Version 5.2019, June 7, 2019).

NCCN Foundation® seeks to support the millions of patients and their families affected by a cancer diagnosis by funding and distributing NCCN Guidelines for Patients®. NCCN Foundation is also committed to advancing cancer treatment by funding the nation's promising doctors at the center of innovation in cancer research. For more details and the full library of patient and caregiver resources, visit NCCN.org/patients. We rely solely on donations to fund the NCCN Guidelines for Patients. To donate, visit NCCNFoundation.org/Donate.

National Comprehensive Cancer Network® (NCCN®) and NCCN Foundation®
3025 Chemical Road, Suite 100 | Plymouth Meeting, PA 19462 | 215.690.0300

Endorsed by

American Lung Association
The American Lung Association strongly supports efforts to help ensure all patients facing lung cancer get the highest standard of treatment and care. Helping patients understand treatment guidelines is one important step in empowering them to get the care they want and need. That is why we are pleased to endorse NCCN's efforts to provide accessible treatment guidelines and information to patients through the NCCN Guidelines for Patients. Lung.org

Bonnie J. Addario Lung Cancer Foundation
The Bonnie J. Addario Lung Cancer Foundation is proud to endorse these NCCN Guidelines for Patients. We believe that educated and empowered patients live longer. This book should be in the hands of every patient diagnosed with lung cancer. lungcancerfoundation.org

Caring Ambassadors
The Caring Ambassador Lung Cancer Program is pleased to endorse these NCCN Guidelines for Patients: Lung Cancer. Patients and their loved ones need reliable resources to achieve the best possible outcomes for their disease. lungcancercap.org

Dusty Joy Foundation (LiveLung)
With patients' best interest at heart, NCCN defines the standard of care for patients and physicians through proven scientific methods and expectations for new discoveries leading to improved patient outcomes. As a lung cancer advocacy nonprofit, our organization wholeheartedly supports the NCCN Guidelines for Patients. LiveLung.org

Free ME from Lung Cancer
As a lung cancer survivor and President and CEO of Free ME from Lung Cancer, I am pleased to endorse this vitally important resource so that lung cancer patients can have the information needed to make informed decisions about their treatment. freeMEfromLungCancer.org

Lung Cancer Action Network (LungCAN)
The NCCN provides the most current standards for patient care in an easy-to-understand and highly accessible format. As a collaborative association of approximately 25 U.S.-based nonprofits dedicated to lung cancer, the Lung Cancer Action Network (LungCAN) is proud to endorse NCCN Guidelines for Patients®: Lung Cancer. LungCAN.org

Lung Cancer Alliance
Lung Cancer Alliance is proud to collaborate with the National Comprehensive Cancer Network to endorse these NCCN Guidelines for Patients®: Lung Cancer. lungcanceralliance.org

Lung Cancer Circle of Hope
Lung Cancer Circle of Hope (LCCH) emphatically endorses the NCCN Guidelines for Patients. Knowledge is power and with this comprehensive resource, patients and their families can proactively work with a qualified physician to make informed decisions in the battle to conquer cancer. lungcancercircleofhope.org

Lung Cancer Initiative of North Carolina
As an organization specializing in connecting patients, survivors and loved ones with the medical research community, the Lung Cancer Initiative of NC fully supports these NCCN Guidelines for Patients. These guidelines set the standard for patient education and access to care. lungcancerinitiativenc.org

Lung Cancer Research Foundation
As a non-profit organization focused on supporting lung cancer research, the Lung Cancer Research Foundation is proud to endorse the NCCN guidelines. These guidelines play an important role in providing lung cancer patients with up to date information and empowering them to make informed decisions about their care. lcrf.org

LUNGevity Foundation
LUNGevity Foundation supports the NCCN Guidelines for Patients as an excellent resource, as we strongly believe in providing education for all those affected by the disease. LUNGevity.org

Special thank you to

Kristina Gregory
Chia-Lin Hung
Wasim Khan
Betty Tong

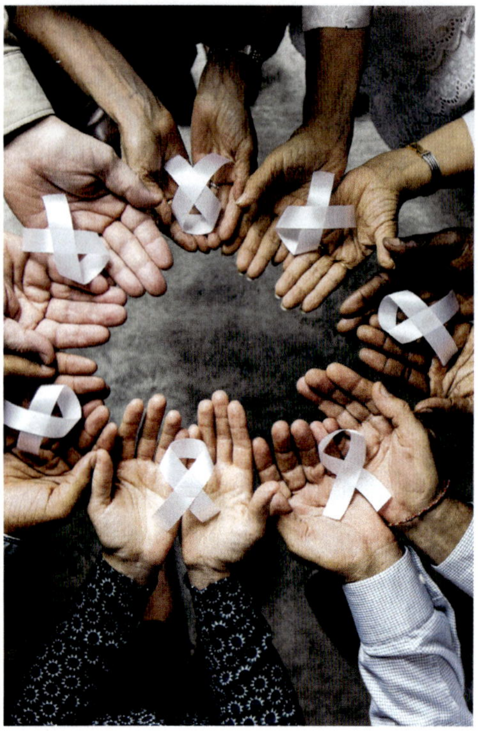
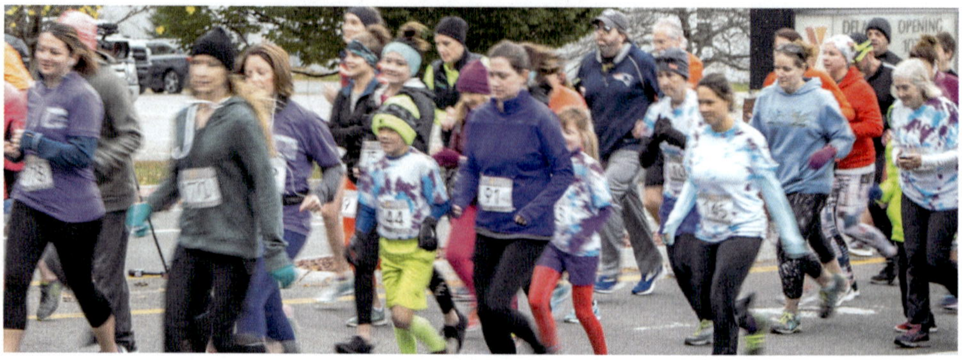
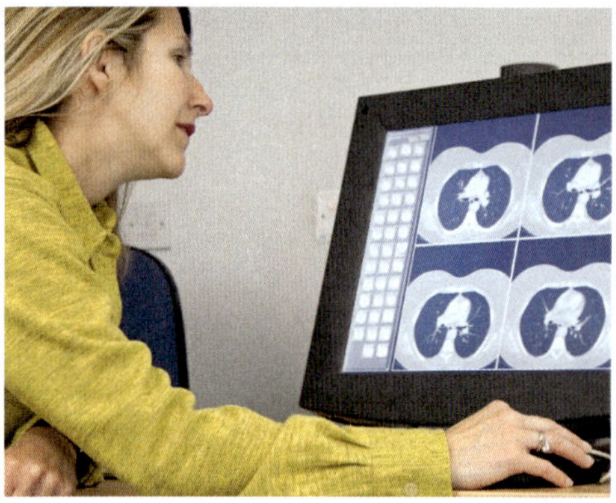
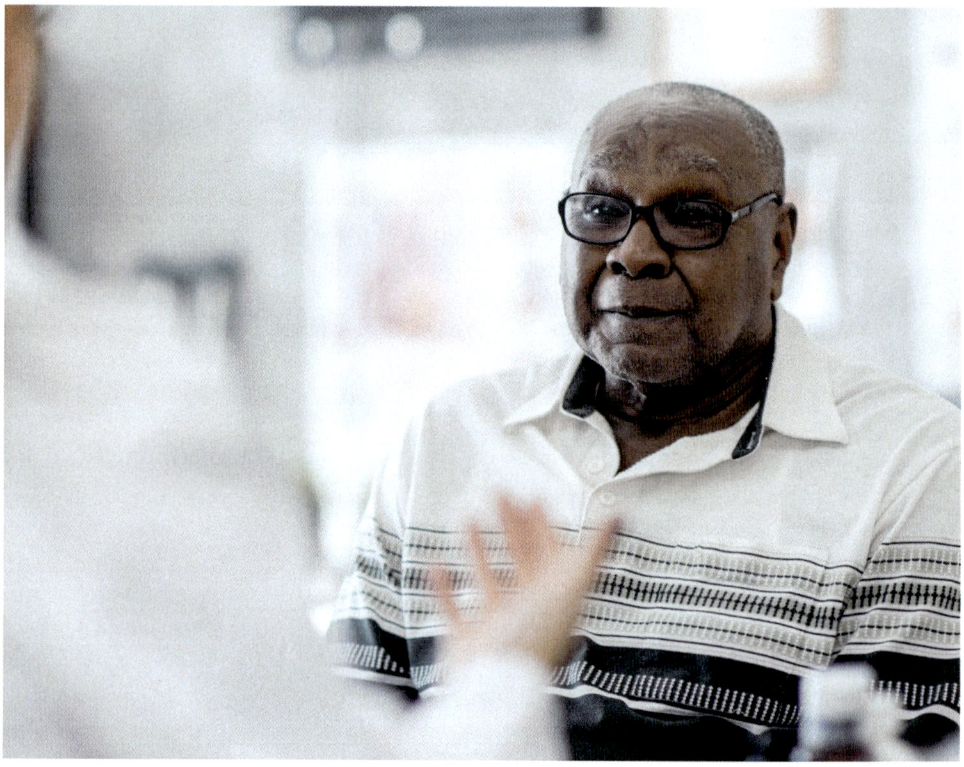
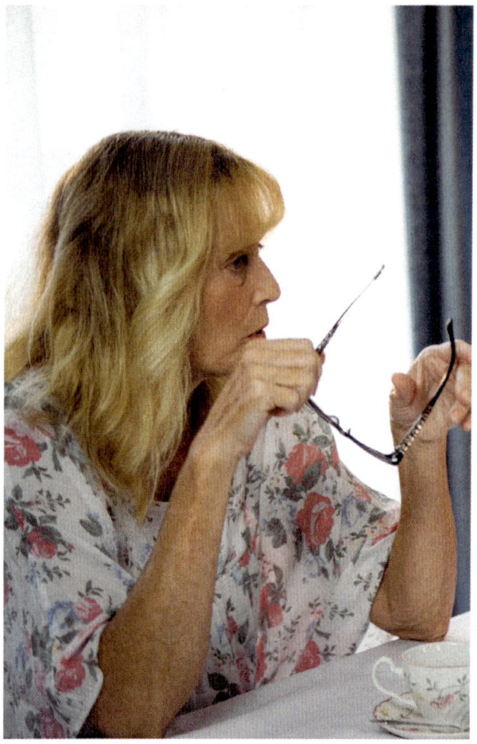
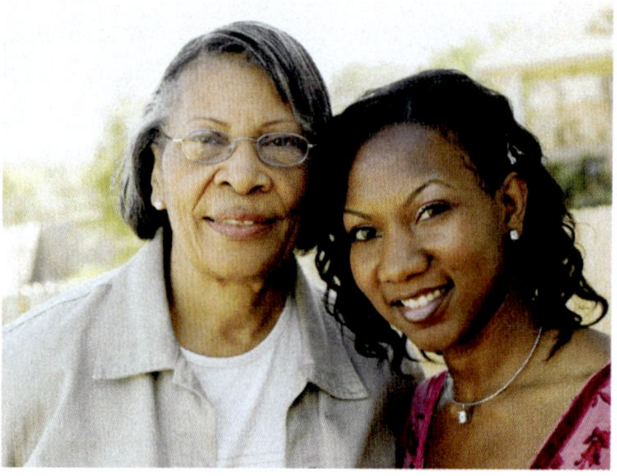
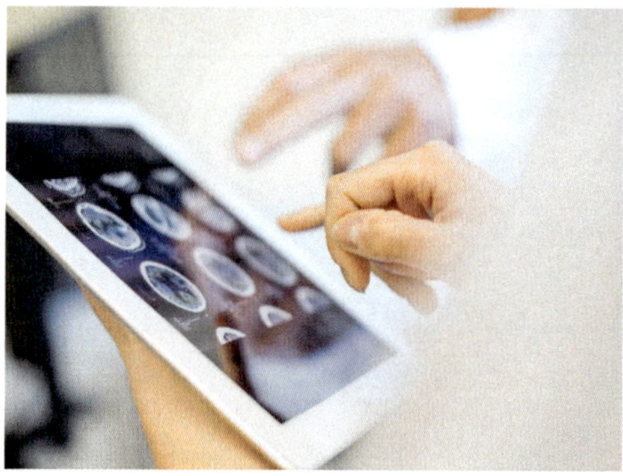
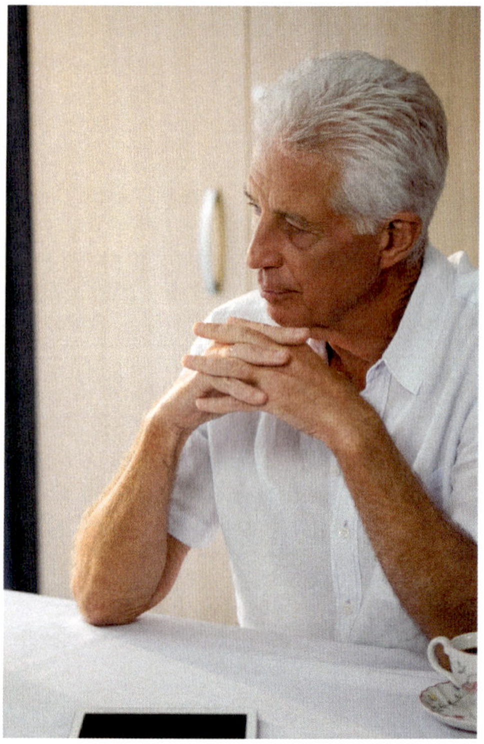

Contents

1
Lung cancer basics

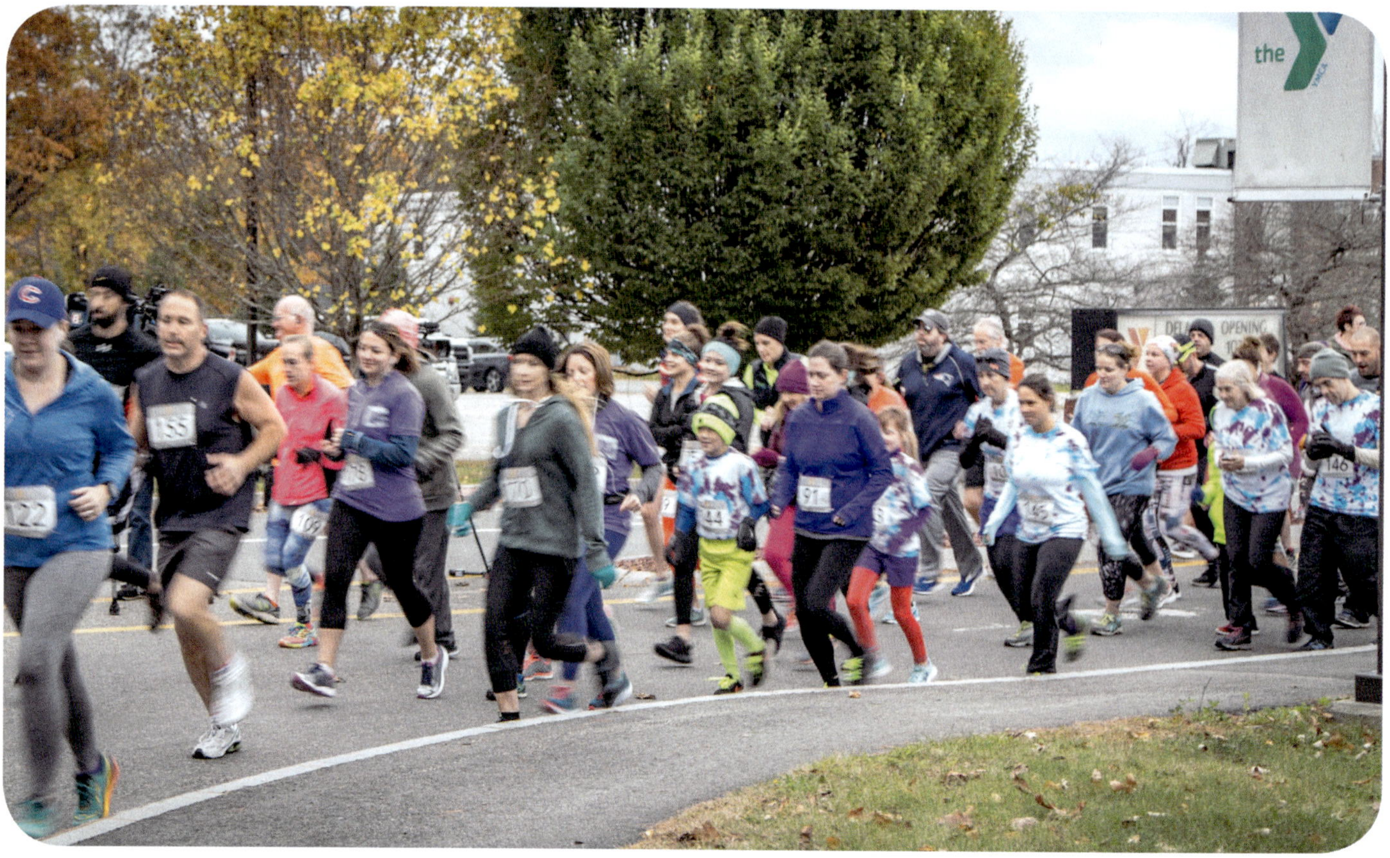

You've learned that you have or may have lung cancer. It's common to feel shocked and confused. This chapter reviews some basics that may help you learn about lung cancer.

Lungs

To learn about lung cancer, you first must know about the lungs. The lungs are the main organs of the respiratory system. They are involved in the exchange of gases in and out of the body.

Airways

Your lungs transfer oxygen—a gas that cells need to live—from the air into the blood. The blood then carries oxygen to all the cells in the body. The lungs also remove carbon dioxide—a gas made by cells—from the blood. Carbon dioxide is then exhaled from the lungs into the air. The transfer of these gases in and out of the body is called respiration.

When you inhale, air travels down your throat into your windpipe (trachea). **See Figure 1**. Air then enters your lungs through the bronchi. The bronchi branch off into each part (lobe) of your lung. Your right lung has three lobes and your left lung has only two lobes to make space for your heart.

Within the lobes, the bronchi divide into smaller airways called bronchioli. At the end of each bronchioli are bunches of alveoli wrapped in blood vessels. The transfer of gases in and out of the blood occurs in the alveoli.

Figure 1
The airways and lungs

Oxygen enters your body through a series of airways that include the windpipe (trachea), bronchi, and bronchioli. Inside your lungs, oxygen is transferred into the bloodstream in the alveoli. Carbon dioxide is transferred out of the bloodstream in the alveoli and exits your body through your airways.

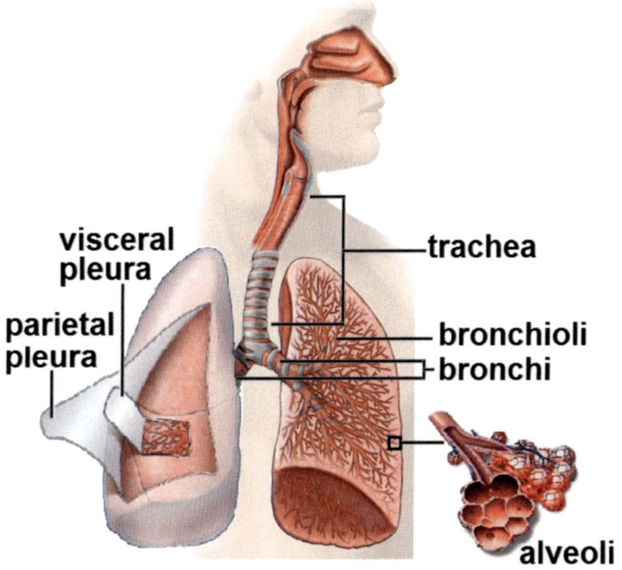

Lymph

Throughout your body—including in your lungs—is a clear fluid called lymph. Lymph gives cells food and water. It also contains germ-fighting immune cells. Lymph drains from tissue into vessels that transport it to the bloodstream. **See Figure 2**. As lymph travels, it passes through small structures called lymph nodes. Lymph nodes remove germs from lymph.

Pleura

Your lungs are protected by tissue called the pleura. Pleura covers each lung and helps the lungs safely rub against other organs. Pleura is made of two layers. The outer layer is known as the parietal pleura. The inner layer is called the visceral pleura. The space in between the two layers is called the pleural cavity. It is filled with a small amount of fluid called pleural fluid.

A disease of cells

Your body is made of trillions of cells. Cancer is a disease of cells. Each type of cancer is named after the cell from which it formed.

Lung cancer

Lung cancer starts in cells of the lung. Other cancers that have spread to the lung are not lung cancers. For example, breast cancer that has spread to the lungs is still breast cancer.

Almost all lung cancers are carcinomas. Carcinomas are cancers of cells that line the inner or outer surfaces of the body. Lung carcinomas start in cells that line the airways of the lungs.

NSCLC

Lung carcinomas are divided into two groups based on how the cells look. One group is called small cell lung cancer and the other group is called NSCLC (**n**on-**s**mall **c**ell **l**ung **c**ancer). The second group is much more common and is the focus of this book.

There are two major types of NSCLC. The first type is non-squamous carcinoma. It includes adenocarcinomas, large-cell carcinomas, and rare cell types. The second type of NSCLC is squamous cell carcinoma. It is also sometimes called epidermoid carcinoma.

Mutations

Cells have a control center called the nucleus. The nucleus contains chromosomes, which are long strands of DNA (**d**eoxyribo**n**ucleic **a**cid) tightly wrapped around proteins. **See Figure 3**. Within DNA are coded instructions for building new cells and controlling how cells behave. These instructions are called genes.

There can be abnormal changes in genes called mutations. Some types of mutations that are linked to cancer are present in all cells. Other mutations are present only in cancer cells. Mutations cause cancer cells to not behave like normal cells and, sometimes, to look very different from normal cells.

Figure 2
Lymph vessels and nodes

Throughout your body, including your lungs, is a network of vessels that transport lymph to the bloodstream. Lymph is a clear fluid that contains germ-fighting blood cells. As lymph travels in vessels, it passes through lymph nodes, which remove germs from lymph.

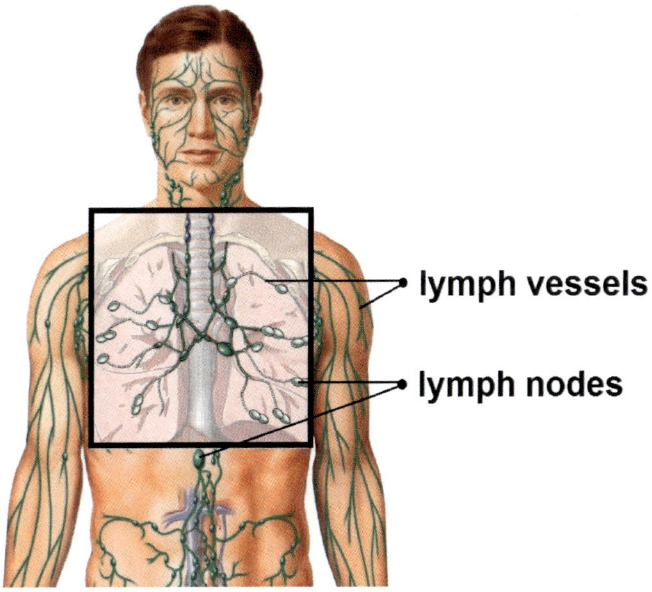

Figure 3
Genetic material in cells

Most human cells contain a plan called the "blueprint of life." It is a plan for how our bodies are made and work. It is found inside of chromosomes. Chromosomes are long strands of DNA that are tightly wrapped around proteins. Genes are small pieces of DNA. Humans have about 20,000 to 25,000 genes.

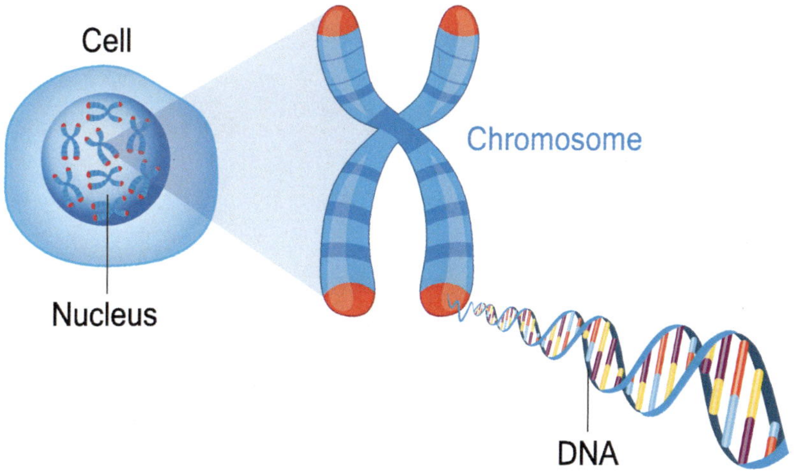

Cancer's threat

When needed, normal cells grow and then divide to form new cells. When old or damaged, they die as shown in **Figure 4**. Normal cells also stay in place. Cancer cells don't behave like normal cells. Cancer cells differ from normal cells in three key ways.

Mass of cells

Cancer cells make new cells that aren't needed. They don't die quickly when old or damaged. Over time, cancer cells form a mass called the primary tumor.

Invasion

The second way cancer cells differ from normal cells is that they can grow into surrounding tissues. If not treated, the primary tumor can grow through an airway. It can even grow into nearby structures. This is called invasion. Lung cancer can invade another bronchus or the pleura. Cancer cells can replace many normal cells making it hard to breathe.

Metastasis

Third, unlike normal cells, cancer cells can leave the lungs. This process is called metastasis. In this process, cancer cells break away from the tumor and merge with blood or lymph. Then, the cancer cells travel in blood or lymph through vessels to other sites. Once in other sites, cancer cells may form secondary tumors and cause major health problems.

> "A major mass in my left lung was found but no tumors elsewhere. I was told it was stage 4 because the pleural effusion fluid tested positive for cancer cells. Then, I developed bilateral embolisms in my lungs.
>
> – Fred
> Lung cancer survivor

Figure 4
Normal cells vs. cancer cells

Normal cells increase in number when they are needed and die when old or damaged. In contrast, cancer cells quickly make new cells and live longer because of abnormal changes in genes.

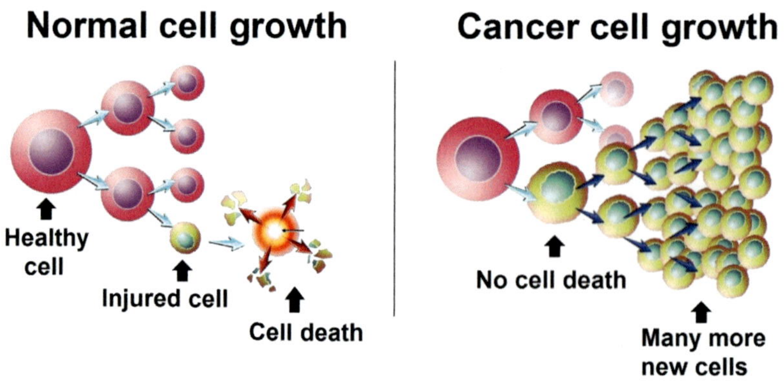

Cancer stages

A cancer stage describes the extent of the cancer in the body. Your doctor uses it for many things. It is used to assess the outlook of the cancer (prognosis). It is used to plan treatment. It is also used for research.

Your doctors may try to diagnose and stage the cancer at the same time. The body part that likely has cancer and is furthest from the lung tumor will be tested. By doing this, you'll have fewer procedures.

For some people, cancer staging is done twice. The rating before any treatment is called the clinical stage. The second staging is called the pathologic stage. It is based on tests of tissue removed during surgery. Sometimes, cancer outside of the lungs isn't found until after surgery.

Staging system

The AJCC (**A**merican **J**oint **C**ommittee on **C**ancer) staging system is used to stage lung cancer. In this system, the letters T, N, and M describe different areas of cancer growth. Your doctors will assign a score to each letter.

The T score tells how large or where the primary tumor has grown. The N score reflects how far lung cancer has spread within nearby lymph nodes. The M scores tells if the cancer has spread to body parts distant from the lung in which it started.

Numbered stages

The TNM scores will be combined to assign the cancer a stage. The stages of lung cancer range from stage 0 to stage 4. Occult carcinoma is also included. Doctors write these stages as—stage 0, stage I, stage II, stage III, and stage IV.

Occult carcinoma

Occult carcinoma means a primary tumor was not found. Lung cancer cells may have been found in fluids or mucus from the lungs. There are no signs of lung cancer in other parts of the body.

Stage 0

Stage 0 means there are abnormal or cancer cells in airways. The cancer cells haven't grown into lung tissue or spread outside the lung.

Stages I–III

Stages I through III have grown into lung tissue. Some have spread to nearby lymph nodes. They have not spread to body parts far from the primary tumor.

Stage IV

Metastatic lung cancers have spread to body parts far from the primary tumor. Stage IV is metastatic cancer that was present at diagnosis. Over time, other stages of lung cancer may metastasize. Lung cancer tends to spread to the brain, adrenal gland, and to the lung without the primary tumor.

Snapshot: Metastatic lung cancer

- ✓ Has spread to body parts far from the lung in which it started
- ✓ Often occurs in the other lung, brain, bone, liver, and adrenal gland
- ✓ When present at diagnosis is rated stage IV
- ✓ Includes earlier stages of lung cancer that have spread far after diagnosis

Treatment types

Not everyone with metastatic lung cancer receives the same treatment. Your doctor will tailor treatment to you based on tests described in **Part 2**. Your treatment will partly depend on the number of metastases.

Local treatment

Local treatment may be an option if metastases are limited. Examples include one tumor in the non-primary lung or cancer spread to only the brain or adrenal gland. Local treatments may also be used to reduce (palliate) symptoms caused by a metastasis.

Local treatment includes surgery, radiation therapy, and chemoradiation. More then one type of local treatment may be used. If needed, the pleural fluid may be drained or the two pleural layers fused.

Systemic treatment

Most often, local treatment is not the main option for metastatic lung cancer. Instead, systemic therapy is often used for cancer control. Systemic therapy affects all cancer in the body. Medical oncologists are cancer doctors trained to use systemic therapy. Options for systemic therapy are presented in **Part 3**.

Clinical trial

One treatment choice may be whether to join a clinical trial. Joining a clinical trial is strongly supported. NCCN believes that you will receive the best management in a clinical trial.

A clinical trial is a type of research that studies a test or treatment in people. It gives people access to health care that otherwise couldn't usually be received. Ask your treatment team if there is an open clinical trial that you can join.

Review

- The lungs help the body get the air it needs to live.
- The lungs are made of many small airways and sacs.
- Lung cancer often starts in the cells that line the airways. These cancers are called carcinomas.
- Cancer cells form a tumor since they don't grow and die as normal cells do.
- Cancer cells can spread to other body parts through lymph or blood.
- Metastatic lung cancer has spread to body parts far from the lung in which it started.
- Treatment partly depends on the number of metastases.
- Clinical trials give people access to new tests and treatments that they otherwise couldn't have received.

2
Treatment planning

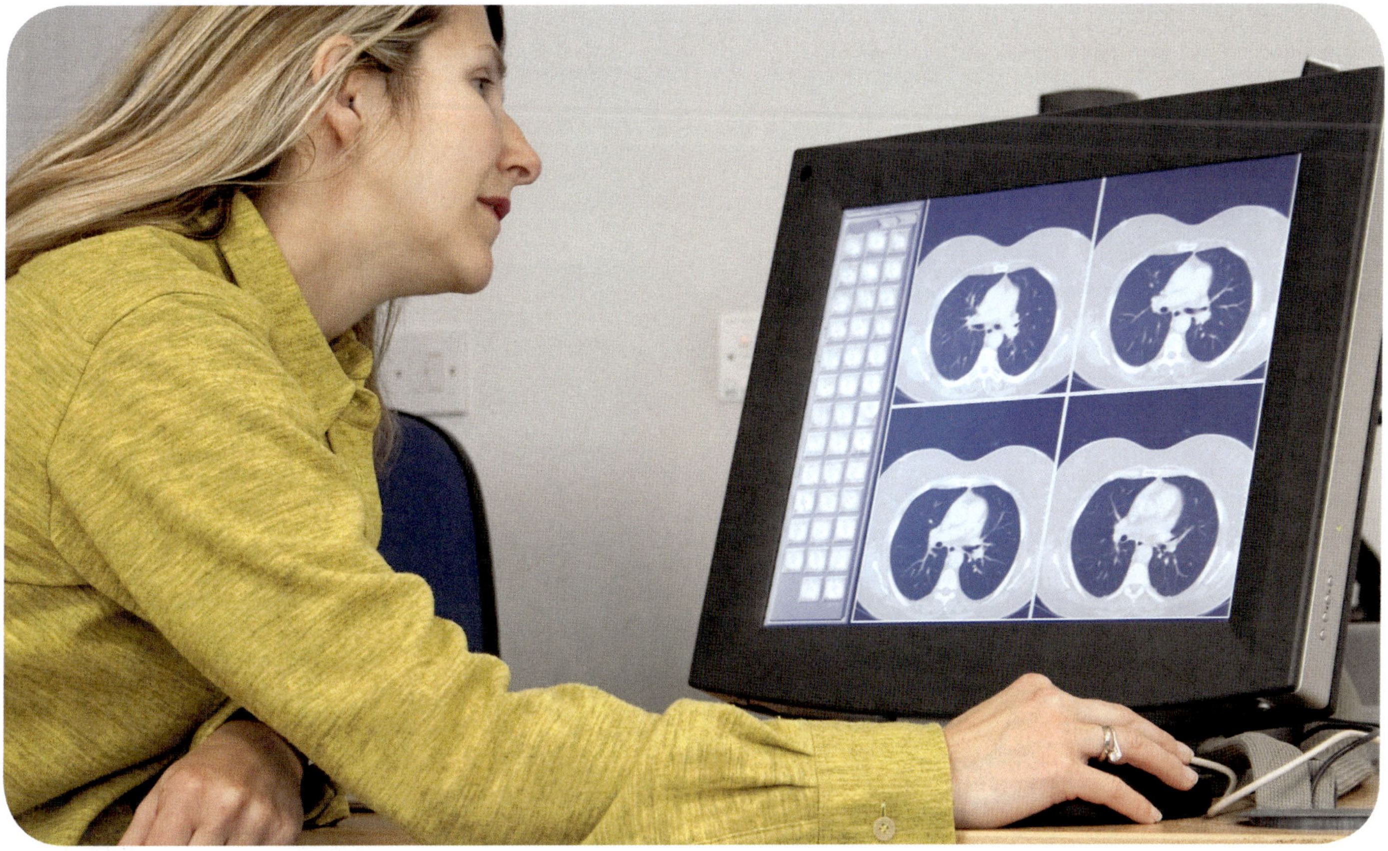

Not all lung cancers are the same. Your doctors will want to learn all about the cancer you have. This chapter describes what health care should be received before treatment.

Doctors plan treatment using many sources of information. These sources include the health care listed in Guide 1. Another source is you. Tell your doctor your concerns and goals for treatment. Together, you can share in the decision-making process. Read **Part 4** to learn more about making treatment decisions.

Guide 1. Health care before cancer treatment

Tests and services
Medical history
Physical exam
Smoking treatment as needed
CBC
Chemistry profile
Diagnostic CT of chest and upper abdomen
FDG PET/CT as needed
Brain MRI
Biopsy
For lung adenocarcinomas, large-cell lung carcinomas, and unknown subtypes: • *EGFR* testing • *ALK* testing • *ROS1* testing • *BRAF* testing • PD-L1 testing
For squamous cell carcinomas: • *EGFR*, *ALK*, *ROS1*, or *BRAF* testing for some people • PD-L1 testing for everyone
Lung function tests as needed
Supportive care

Medical history

Your doctor will ask about any health problems and treatment you have had in your life. Be prepared to list your illnesses and injuries. You will also be asked about health conditions and symptoms. It may help to bring a list of old and new medicines to your doctor's office.

Your doctor will ask about symptoms that may be related to lung cancer. Such symptoms include cough, trouble breathing, chest pain, and weight loss. Knowing which symptoms you have can help your doctors stage the cancer.

Some cancers and other health conditions can run in families. Thus, your doctor will ask about the medical history of your close blood relatives. Such family members include your siblings, parents, and grandparents. Be prepared to tell who has had what diseases and at what ages.

Your doctor will ask if you have ever smoked. Tell him or her if you smoke or have smoked in the past. You'll also be asked how much you've smoked in your lifetime. Smoking is often measured by packs per day and the number of years that you have smoked.

Physical exam

A physical exam is a study of your body. It is done to look for signs of disease. It is also used to help assess what treatments may be options.

To start, your basic body functions will be measured. These functions include your temperature, blood pressure, and pulse and breathing rate. Your weight will also be checked.

Your doctor will listen to your lungs, heart, and gut. He or she will also assess your eyes, skin, nose, ears, and mouth. Parts of your body will be felt. Your doctor will note the size of organs and if they feel soft or hard. Tell your doctor if you feel pain when touched.

Your doctor will also rate your performance status. Performance status is your ability to do daily activities. It is used by doctors to assess if you can undergo certain treatments. Read **Part 3** for more information.

Smoking treatment

If you smoke, it is important to quit. Smoking can limit how well cancer treatment works. Nicotine addiction is one of the hardest addictions to stop. The stress of having cancer may make it harder to quit. There is help. Ask your doctor about counseling and drugs to help you quit.

Blood tests

Lung cancer is not found in blood. Instead, doctors test blood to look for signs of disease. Blood tests require a sample of your blood. Blood samples can be removed with a blood draw.

Blood draw

Some blood draws require no eating and drinking for hours. Your doctor will say if you can eat or drink. Blood samples will be removed with a needle placed into your vein.

Your blood will be tested by a pathologist. A pathologist is a doctor who's an expert in testing tissue and cells. He or she will send the lab results to your doctor.

Complete blood count

A CBC (**c**omplete **b**lood **c**ount) measures parts of the blood. This lab test gives a picture of your overall health. Test results include counts of white blood cells, red blood cells, and platelets. Cancer and other health problems can cause low or high counts.

Chemistry profile

Chemicals in your blood come from your liver, bone, and other organs. A chemistry profile assesses if the chemicals in your blood are too low or high. Abnormal levels can be caused by spread of cancer or by other health problems.

Imaging

Imaging makes pictures of the insides of your body. It can show which body parts have cancer. Some types of imaging also reveal some features of a tumor and its cells. A radiologist is a doctor who is an expert in reading images. He or she will convey the test results to your doctor.

Your treatment team will tell you what to expect for these tests. You may need to stop taking some medicines and stop eating and drinking for a few hours before the scan. Tell your doctors if you get nervous when in small spaces. See **Figure 5**. You may be given a pill to help you relax.

Some imaging uses contrast. Contrast is a dye that makes the pictures clearer. Tell your doctor if you've had problems with contrast in the past.

Diagnostic CT

Diagnostic CT (**c**omputed **t**omography) should be one of the first tests used for cancer staging. It uses higher doses of radiation than low-dose CT. As a result, the images show more details. Contrast should be used.

For cancer staging, imaging of your chest and upper abdomen is needed. Your doctor will use the results to plan where to biopsy and which treatment is best. For example, your doctor may biopsy your adrenal gland if a mass is found with CT.

FDG PET/CT

CT may be combined with PET (**p**ositron **e**mission **t**omography). When used together, they are called a PET/CT scan. This scan is sometimes given when lung cancer is stage IV. It may find cancer not found by CT alone.

A FDG (**f**luoro**d**eoxy**g**lucose) radiotracer will be used. Cancer quickly uses glucose so it appears "hot" in images. Other health problems can also cause hot spots, too. Cancer detected by PET/CT often needs to be confirmed with biopsy or other imaging.

Brain MRI

MRI (**m**agnetic **r**esonance **i**maging) is an imaging test that uses a magnetic field and radio waves. If you have or may have metastatic lung cancer, brain MRI is very important. It will show if the cancer has spread to your brain.

Figure 5
CT machine

Pictures of the insides of your body can be made with imaging. During the scan, you will lie on a table that will move into the tunnel of the machine. The pictures will be viewed by a doctor who will look for signs of cancer.

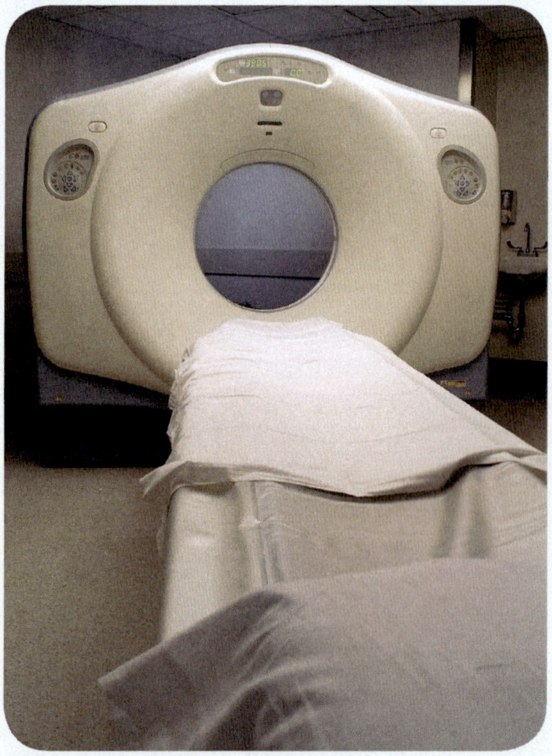

Biopsy

A biopsy is a procedure that removes tissue or fluid samples for testing. If tests suggest metastasis, a biopsy is needed before treatment. Often, the metastasis is biopsied instead of the primary tumor.

Your doctor will use imaging results to select the biopsy site. This site is often the adrenal gland, liver, or bone. The type of biopsy that will be done depends on the site.

- **External needle biopsies** involve guiding a thin needle through your skin and into the tumor. These biopsies include TTNA (**t**rans**t**horacic **n**eedle **a**spiration), core needle biopsies, pericardiocentesis, and thoracentesis.
- **Down-the-throat biopsies** involve guiding tools down your throat into your windpipe or esophagus. These biopsies include bronchoscopy and EUS (**e**ndoscopic **u**ltra**s**ound)-guided biopsies.
- **Portal surgeries** involve cutting small holes (ports) into your chest. Small tools are inserted through the ports to remove tissue. Compared to open surgery, this technique is "minimally invasive." These surgeries include thoracoscopy.
- **Open surgery** involves making a large cut into your skin to remove tissue. You may have open surgery when other methods won't work or a larger piece of tissue is needed.

Ask your doctor

Will the biopsy remove a large enough sample for biomarker (molecular) testing?

Cancer lab tests

Not all lung cancers are alike. Lung cancer differs between people. A pathologist will study the tissue or fluid samples from your body. If cancer is confirmed, more lab tests will be done to learn about the cancer.

All lab results are included in a pathology report. This report will be sent to your doctor. Ask him or her for a copy. Your doctor will review the results with you. Take notes and ask questions.

Histologic typing

The pathologist will study the parts of the cancer cells to classify the disease. This is called histologic typing. The pathology report will state if the cancer started in the lung or elsewhere. If the cancer started in the lung, the report will also list the type of lung cancer.

Histologic types of NSCLC include squamous cell carcinoma, adenocarcinoma, large-cell lung carcinoma, and other mixed and rare types. Squamous cells are thin and flat and line the airways of the lung. Adenocarcinoma is a cancer of epithelial cells that make fluids to keep the lungs moist. Large-cell lung carcinomas lack features to classify them as any other carcinoma.

Biomarker testing

Lung cancer also differs between people by which markers are present. Biomarker (or molecular) testing looks for these markers. It may include tests of genes or their products (proteins). Results are used to plan treatment.

Most often, biomarker testing is done on tissue samples. Sometimes, a sample of blood may be used for biomarker testing. A blood sample is referred to as a "liquid biopsy."

Overactive EGFR mutations

EGFR (**e**pidermal **g**rowth **f**actor **r**eceptor) is a surface receptor. Surface receptors are structures on the outer membrane of cells. They start changes within a cell when turned on. **See Figure 6**.

Some lung cancers consist of cells with mutations in the gene that controls EGFR. Some of these mutations cause the receptors to be overactive. When overactive, EGFR causes new cancer cells to form quickly.

EGFR mutation testing is advised for certain metastatic lung cancers. It is standard for adenocarcinomas, large-cell lung carcinomas, and unknown subtypes. Very few squamous cell carcinomas have overactive *EGFR* mutations. But, testing may be done if you've never smoked or the cancer has a mixed histology.

"When my biopsy was performed, the tissue was sent off for testing. I have a mutation that allows for targeted therapy. My treatment team is superb!

– Mary
Lung cancer survivor

Figure 6
Surface receptor

Some lung cancers consist of cells with abnormal surface receptors. A surface receptor is a protein on the outer membrane of cells. It starts changes within a cell when turned on. Receptors that may be abnormal and help lung cancer grow include EGFR, ALK, and ROS1.

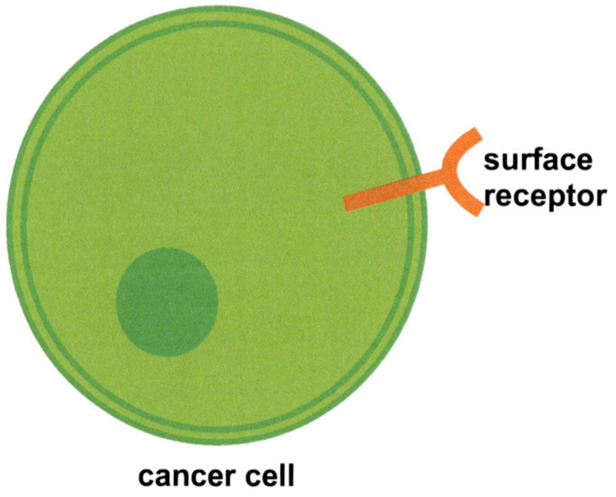

ALK gene rearrangement

ALK (**a**naplastic **l**ymphoma **k**inase) is another type of surface receptor. It can be overactive causing cancer cells to quickly grow. Overactive ALKs occur when there is *ALK* gene rearrangement. A gene rearrangement is the fusion of one gene with another gene to create a new gene.

ALK testing is advised for certain metastatic lung cancers. It is standard for adenocarcinomas, large-cell lung carcinomas, and unknown subtypes. Very few squamous cell carcinomas have *ALK* gene rearrangements. But, testing may be done if you've never smoked or the cancer has a mixed histology.

ROS1 gene rearrangement

ROS1 is a surface receptor that is overactive in a small number of lung cancers. Overactive ROS1s occur when there is *ROS1* gene rearrangement. *ROS1* testing is advised for metastatic lung adenocarcinomas, large-cell lung carcinomas, and unknown subtypes. Sometimes, testing is done for squamous cell carcinomas.

BRAF V600E mutation

BRAF is a signaling protein inside of cells. It is overactive due to a *BRAF* V600E mutation in a small number of lung cancers. *BRAF* testing is advised for metastatic lung adenocarcinomas, large-cell lung carcinomas, and unknown subtypes. Sometimes, testing is done for squamous cell carcinomas.

PD-L1 expression

T cells are part of your body's disease-fighting (immune) system. One job of T cells is to attack cancer cells. Some lung cancers consist of cells that make (express) molecules called PD-L1. PD-L1 attaches to PD-1 on T cells and stops them from attacking cancer cells. All types of metastatic lung cancer should be tested for PD-L1 expression.

Snapshot: Biomarker testing

Not all metastatic lung cancers are alike. They differ by which, if any, markers are present.

- ✓ Testing will help pinpoint which treatments will or won't work.
- ✓ Most lung cancers do not have a marker.
- ✓ Very few squamous cell carcinomas have EGFR, ALK, ROS1, or BRAF markers.
- ✓ Most often, *EGFR*, *ALK*, *ROS1*, and *BRAF* markers do not occur together.
- ✓ All lung cancers should be tested for PD-L1 expression.
- ✓ Broad molecular profiling is advised so rare markers for which there are treatments can be found.

Other biomarkers

There are other known biomarkers linked with NSCLC. However, they are rare and related treatments are still being tested in clinical trials. Testing for these biomarkers should be done along with *EGFR, ALK, ROS1*, and *BRAF* testing. There may be treatments available or a clinical trial you could join. Other gene changes linked with lung cancer include:

- *NTRK* gene fusion,
- High-level *MET* amplification,
- *MET* exon 14 skipping mutation,
- *RET* gene rearrangements,
- *HER2* mutations, and
- Tumor mutational burden.

Lung function tests

Surgery or radiation therapy may be treatment options for some limited stage IV cancers. First, your doctors will need to know how well your lungs work. Three pulmonary function tests may be done.

- **Spirometry** involves blowing into a tube to measure how much air and how fast you breathe.
- A **gas diffusion test** involves breathing in a harmless gas and measuring how much you breathe out. It tells how much oxygen travels from your lungs into your blood.
- **Body plethysmograph** involves sitting in a small room and breathing into a tube. This test measures how much air your lungs can hold and how much air is left in your lungs after you exhale.

Supportive care

Supportive care aims to improve your quality of life. It includes care for health issues caused by cancer or cancer treatment. It is also sometimes called palliative care.

Palliative care is important for everyone, not just people at the end of life. In fact, it has been shown to extend and enhance life for people with metastatic lung cancer.

Treatment side effects

All cancer treatments can cause unwanted health issues. Such health issues are called side effects. Some side effects may be harmful to your health. Others may just be unpleasant.

Side effects depend on many factors. These factors include the treatment type, length or dose of treatment, and the person.

Supportive care can extend and enhance life for people with metastatic lung cancer.

Ask your treatment team for a complete list of side effects of your treatments. Also, tell your treatment team about any new or worse symptoms you get. There may be ways to help you feel better. There are also ways to prevent some side effects.

Review

- A medical history is a report of all health events in your lifetime.
- Your doctor will examine your body for signs of disease. He or she will touch parts of your body to see if anything feels abnormal.
- Ask your doctor for help to quit smoking.
- Blood tests are used to look for signs of cancer.
- Diagnostic CT may show where the cancer has spread in your body. PET/CT may detect cancer that CT did not.
- MRI is used to see if the cancer has spread to your brain.
- A biopsy is needed before treatment. Often, samples from the adrenal gland, liver, or bone are removed.
- Not all lung cancers are the same. Molecular testing can show which, if any, markers are present in lung cancer cells.
- Pulmonary function tests are needed if surgery or radiation therapy is a treatment option.
- Start supportive care early. It has been shown to extend and enhance life for people with metastatic lung cancer.

"

Learning to manage side effects is well worth the effort!

– Jon
Lung cancer survivor

3
Treatment guide

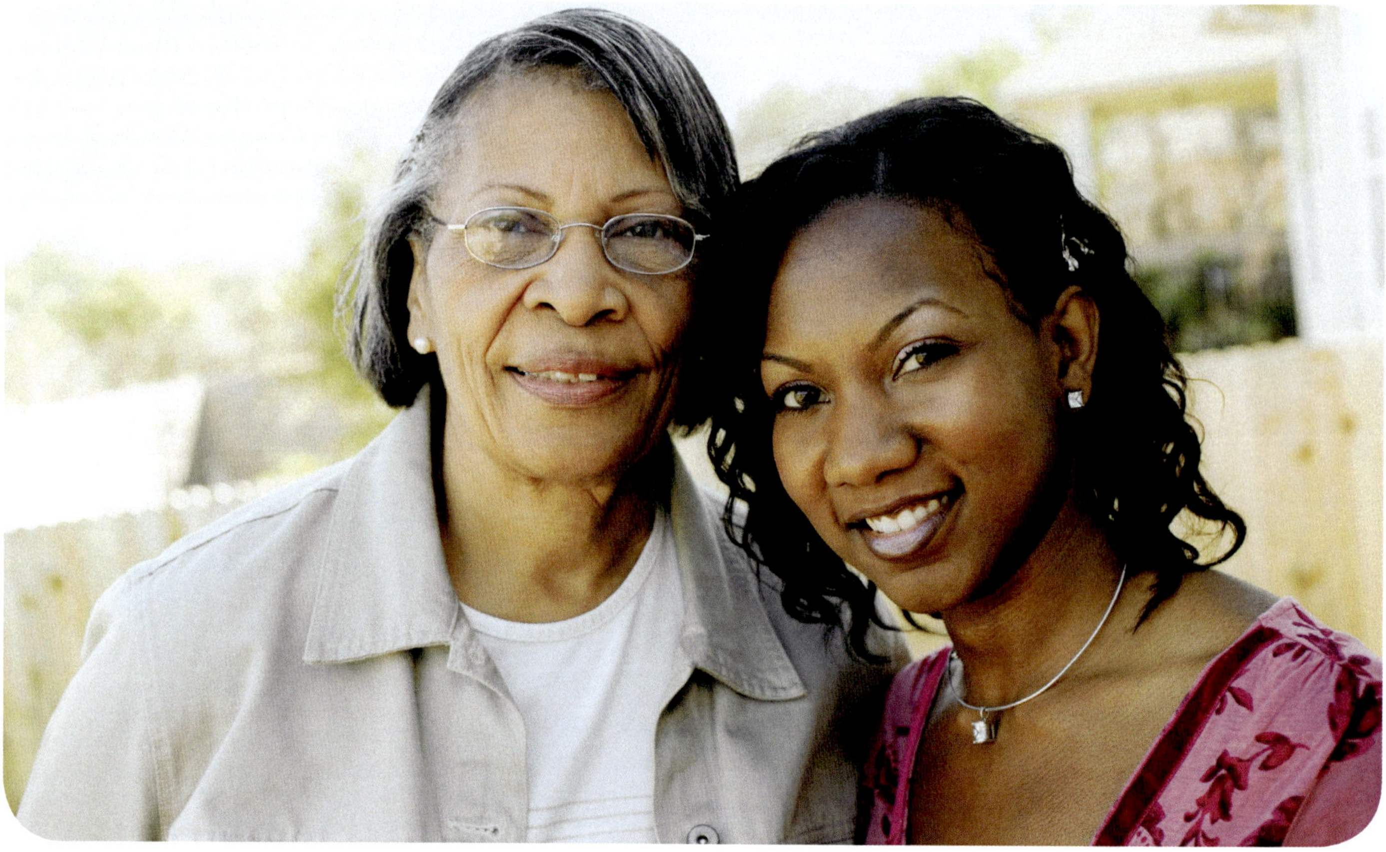

Based on the test results, your treatment can be tailored to you. This chapter presents treatment options based on features of the cancer. Starting supportive care early is also important.

Overview

Treatment of metastatic lung cancer includes treatment of the cancer and support for you. At this time, metastatic lung cancer is unlikely to be cured. Instead, the aim of treatment is to reduce symptoms, control the cancer, and extend life.

Treatment options depend on many factors. One main factor is the presence or absence of biomarkers. If biomarkers are absent or unknown, treatment depends on the type of lung cancer. In this chapter, treatment options are listed by which biomarker is present, if any.

The treatment approach for metastatic cancer is to use one treatment after another. A treatment is used until it stops working or side effects get too bad. Then another treatment is started. This approach is followed until you want to stop or there are no options. Long-term cancer control may be achieved for some people.

First-line treatment is the first treatment(s) given. After 2 cycles, you will get a CT scan to assess treatment results. Contrast may be used. If results are good, you'll get CT scans every 2 to 4 cycles. If the cancer worsens, results of next-in-line treatment are tested every 6 to 12 weeks.

Treatment options

Treatment options depend on the presence or absence of biomarkers. Most lung cancers do not have biomarkers for which there is treatment. Instead, they are treated based on the type of lung cancer.

Overactive *EGFR* mutation

Targeted therapy slows the growth of lung cancer with *EGFR* mutations. The type of targeted therapy that is used is called a tyrosine kinase inhibitor. These drugs attach to a part of EGFR that is within cells. They stop EGFRs from sending signals that tell the cell to grow.

EGFR mutations may be found while you are on first-line chemotherapy. In this case, you may stop chemotherapy early and start targeted therapy. Or, you may start targeted therapy after chemotherapy is finished.

First-line treatment

Guide 2 lists the five drugs that are used for first-line treatment. All have been found to work well in well-designed clinical trials. Osimertinib is preferred because it stops cancer growth for a longer period of time. Your doctor will explain which of the five drugs will likely work best for you. It partly depends on which gene mutations are present.

If treatment results are good, keep taking your medicine. If the cancer worsens, a biopsy may be needed. Biomarker testing may find new mutations that cause cancer cells to resist treatment.

Next-in-line treatment

After months of first-line treatment, lung cancer starts to grow again in most people. If it grows while on erlotinib, afatinib, gefitinib, or dacomitinib, *T790M* testing is advised. A liquid biopsy should be first used. *T790M* is a mutation that often occurs in the *EGFR* gene after taking these drugs. It stops the cancer drugs from working.

If the cancer doesn't worsen much, one option may be to stay on first-line treatment. The cancer may worsen quicker if this treatment is stopped. Local treatment for cancer within a confined area may be added. Such cancers include lung cancer only in the brain or adrenal gland.

After first-line erlotinib, afatinib, gefitinib, or dacomitinib, your options may include osimertinib.

Guide 2. Treatment for overactive *EGFR* mutation

What are first-line options?		What are next-in-line options?
• Osimertinib (preferred)	➡	• Stay on osimertinib ± local treatment • Start treatment for histologic type ◦ Adenocarcinomas, large cell, unknown types (see Guide 8) ◦ Squamous cell carcinoma (see Guide 9)
• Erlotinib • Afatinib • Gefitinib • Dacomitinib	➡	• Stay on first-line treatment ± local treatment • Switch to osimertinib if *T790M* present • Start treatment for histologic type if *T790M* not present ◦ Adenocarcinomas, large cell, unknown types (see Guide 8) ◦ Squamous cell carcinoma (see Guide 9)

T790M must be present. Afatinib with cetuximab may also be an option. Cetuximab stops growth signals from EGFR by attaching to EGFR on the outside of cells. More research is needed to pinpoint whom afatinib with cetuximab helps.

If EGFR-targeted therapy is not likely to help, your doctor may advise other treatment. Read Guide 8 to learn options for adenocarcinoma, large cell, and unknown types. Read Guide 9 to learn options for squamous cell carcinoma.

What to expect: Tryosine kinase inhibitors

- ✓ Tryosine kinase inhibitors are often given when an *EGFR*, *ALK*, *ROS1*, *BRAF*, or *NTRK* marker is present.
- ✓ They are sometimes just called TKIs.
- ✓ They are made as a pill but some are also made as a liquid.
- ✓ Some must be taken on an empty stomach while others can be taken with or without food.
- ✓ Some are taken once a day while others are taken twice a day.
- ✓ Your doctor will decide what dose you need.
- ✓ TKIs can cause side effects. Ask your treatment team for a complete list of rare and common side effects.
- ✓ Tell your doctor if you are pregnant, trying to get pregnant, or are breastfeeding. TKIs may harm babies.

ALK rearrangement

Targeted therapy slows the growth of lung cancer with an *ALK* rearrangement. The type of targeted therapy that is used is called a tyrosine kinase inhibitor. These drugs attach to a part of *ALK* that is within cells. They stop *ALK*s from sending signals that tell the cell to grow.

An *ALK* rearrangement may be found while you are on first-line chemotherapy. In this case, you may stop chemotherapy early and start targeted therapy. Or, you may start targeted therapy after chemotherapy is finished.

First-line treatment

Guide 3 lists the four drugs that are used for first-line treatment. All have been found to work well in well-designed clinical trials. Alectinib is preferred because it better controls cancer growth and extends life more. Brigatinib is a newer drug that hasn't been compared to alectinib. Your doctor will explain which of the four drugs will likely work best for you.

If treatment results are good, keep taking your medicine. If the cancer worsens, a biopsy may be needed. Biomarker testing may find new mutations that cause cancer cells to resist treatment.

Next-in-line treatment

Within a few years on first-line treatment, lung cancer starts to grow again in most people. If the cancer doesn't worsen much, one option may be to stay on first-line treatment. The cancer may worsen quicker if this treatment is stopped. Local treatment for cancer within a confined area may be added. Examples include lung cancer in the brain or adrenal gland.

After taking crizotinib, the other targeted therapies may be options if not taken before. Local treatment for cancer within a confined area may be added.

Guide 3. Treatment for *ALK* rearrangement

What are first-line options?		What are next-in-line options?
• Alectinib (preferred) • Brigatinib • Ceritinib	➔	• Stay on first-line treatment ± local treatment • Switch to lorlatinib • Start treatment for histologic type ◦ Adenocarcinomas, large cell, unknown types (see Guide 8) ◦ Squamous cell carcinoma (see Guide 9)
• Crizotinib	➔	• Stay on crizotinib ± local treatment • Switch to alectinib, brigatinib, or ceritinib ± local treatment ◦ After these treatments, switch to lorlatinib • Start treatment for histologic type ◦ Adenocarcinomas, large cell, unknown types (see Guide 8) ◦ Squamous cell carcinoma (see Guide 9)

Lorlatinib may be an option after alectinib, brigatinib, or ceritinib. It treats lung cancer when new mutations stop the other targeted therapies from working.

If ALK-targeted therapy is not likely to help, your doctor may advise other treatment. Read Guide 8 to learn options for adenocarcinoma, large cell, and unknown types. Read Guide 9 to learn options for squamous cell carcinoma.

“

The people that are truly there for you are your angels!

– Jon
Lung cancer survivor

ROS1 rearrangement

Targeted therapy slows the growth of lung cancer with an *ROS1* rearrangement. The type of targeted therapy that is used is called a tyrosine kinase inhibitor. These drugs attach to a part of ROS1 that is within cells. They stop ROS1 from sending signals that tell the cell to grow.

An *ROS1* rearrangement may be found while you are on first-line chemotherapy. In this case, you may stop chemotherapy early and start targeted therapy. Or, you may start targeted therapy after chemotherapy is finished.

First-line treatment

Guide 4 lists the two drugs that are used for first-line treatment. Crizotinib is the preferred option as it controls cancer growth very well. The other option is ceritinib. Your doctor will explain which one will likely work best for you.

If treatment results are good, keep taking your medicine. If the cancer worsens, a biopsy may be needed. Biomarker testing may find new mutations that cause cancer cells to resist treatment.

Next-in-line treatment

Within a few years on first-line treatment, lung cancer starts to grow again in most people. Research is needed to learn if ceritinib is helpful after crizotinib stops working. Lorlatinib may be an option after crizotinib or ceritinib. It treats lung cancer when new mutations stop the other targeted therapies from working.

If ROS1-targeted therapy is not likely to help, your doctor may advise other treatment. Read Guide 8 to learn options for adenocarcinoma, large cell, and unknown types. Read Guide 9 to learn options for squamous cell carcinoma.

Guide 4. Treatment for *ROS1* rearrangement

What are first-line options?	What are next-in-line options?
• Crizotinib (preferred) • Ceritinib	• Switch to lorlatinib • Start treatment for histologic type ◦ Adenocarcinomas, large cell, unknown types (see Guide 8) ◦ Squamous cell carcinoma (see Guide 9)

BRAF V600E mutation

Targeted therapy is one of the options for lung cancer with a *BRAF* V600E mutation. Options are listed in Guide 5. Dabrafenib and trametinib are targeted therapies called tyrosine kinase inhibitors.

BRAF and MEK are proteins within the same signaling pathway. Dabrafenib stops growth signals from BRAF. Trametinib stops growth signals from MEK. If these drugs make you too sick, you may receive dabrafenib or vemurafenib alone. Vemurafenib also stops growth signals from BRAF.

Chemotherapy-based treatment is another option. It may be used for first-line treatment or when targeted therapy stops working. Read Guide 8 to learn options for adenocarcinoma, large cell, and unknown types. Read Guide 9 to learn options for squamous cell carcinoma.

Guide 5. Treatment for *BRAF* V600E mutation

What are the options?
• Dabrafenib + trametinib
• Start treatment for histologic type ◦ Adenocarcinomas, large cell, unknown types (see Guide 8) ◦ Squamous cell carcinoma (see Guide 9)

NTRK gene fusion

Larotrectinib is a newer cancer drug for lung cancer. As listed in Guide 6, it may be an option for metastatic lung cancer with an *NTRK* gene fusion. *NTRK* gene fusions in lung cancer are rare.

Larotrectinib is a targeted therapy called a tyrosine kinase inhibitor. It stops TRK from sending signals that tell the cell to grow.

Chemotherapy-based treatment is another option. It may be used for first-line treatment or when targeted therapy stops working. Read Guide 8 to learn options for adenocarcinoma, large cell, and unknown types. Read Guide 9 to learn options for squamous cell carcinoma.

Guide 6. Treatment for *NTRK* gene fusion

What are the options?
• Larotrectinib
• Start treatment for histologic type ◦ Adenocarcinomas, large cell, unknown types (see Guide 8) ◦ Squamous cell carcinoma (see Guide 9)

PD-L1 ≥1%

Immunotherapy slows the growth of lung cancer with high amounts of PD-L1. A cutoff of ≥1% is used by doctors to decide whom immunotherapy might help. But, levels just below the cutoff will likely have a response like cancers just above the cutoff.

Immunotherapy

The type of immunotherapy that is used is called immune checkpoint inhibitors. PD-1 inhibitors attach to PD-1 on T cells. **See Figure 7**. PD-L1 inhibitors attach to PD-L1 on cancer cells. These inhibitors stop cancer cells with PD-L1 from attaching to T cells. The T cells are then able to attack cancer cells.

Not all lung cancers with high PD-L1 should be treated with immunotherapy. Immunotherapy is of no help if certain cancer-promoting mutations are present. An example is an activating *EGFR* mutation. Immunotherapy may also not be given if it could impair your immune system. Tell your doctor if you have an autoimmune disease, such as Crohn's disease, ulcerative colitis, or lupus.

Figure 7
Immunotherapy

Some lung cancers consist of cells that have PD-L1 on their surface. PD-L1 can attach to T cells and stop them from attacking cancer cells. Immunotherapy for lung cancer stops PD-L1 from attaching. As a result, T cells are able to attack cancer cells.

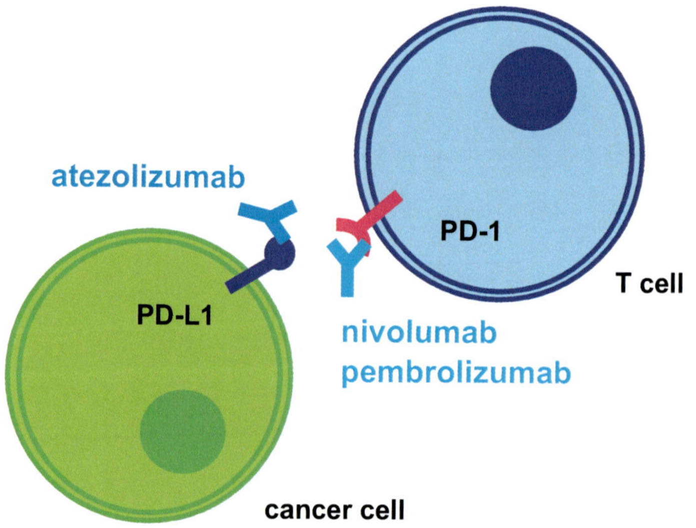

First-line treatment

Guide 7 lists the regimens that are used for first-line treatment. All have been shown to work well in well-designed clinical trials. Pembrolizumab is a PD-1 inhibitor. Used alone, it is the preferred option as it controls cancer growth with fewer side effects. Another option is pembrolizumab with chemotherapy.

There is a third treatment option for adenocarcinomas, large cell, and unknown types. It consists of a PD-L1 inhibitor called atezolizumab as well as chemotherapy and bevacizumab. Bevacizumab is a targeted therapy that stops the growth of blood vessels to tumors. Tumors then don't get the blood they need to survive.

First-line treatment may stop the cancer from getting worse. In this case, you may stay on some of your first-line treatments. This is called maintenance therapy. An example is pembrolizumab with pemetrexed. Another option is to watch and wait (observation).

Next-in-line treatment

Within a few years on first-line treatment, lung cancer starts to grow again in most people. Read Guide 8 to learn options for adenocarcinoma, large cell, and unknown types. Read Guide 9 to learn options for squamous cell carcinoma.

Guide 7. Treatment for PD-L1 ≥1%

Adenocarcinomas, large cell, and unknown types

What are first-line options?	What are next-in-line options?
• Pembrolizumab (preferred if PD-L1 is ≥50%) • (Carboplatin or cisplatin) + pemetrexed + pembrolizumab (preferred if PD-L1 is between 1% and 49%) • Carboplatin + paclitaxel + bevacizumab + atezolizumab	• Start treatment for histologic type ◦ Adenocarcinomas, large cell, unknown types (see Guide 8) ◦ Squamous cell carcinoma (see Guide 9)

Squamous cell carcinoma

What are first-line options?	What are next-in-line options?
• Pembrolizumab (preferred if PD-L1 is ≥50%) • (Carboplatin or cisplatin) + paclitaxel + pembrolizumab (preferred if PD-L1 is between 1% and 49%)	• Start treatment for histologic type ◦ Adenocarcinomas, large cell, unknown types (see Guide 8) ◦ Squamous cell carcinoma (see Guide 9)

Biomarkers are absent or unknown

This section discusses treatment for when biomarkers are absent or unknown. These treatments may also be used after first-line treatment for metastatic lung cancers with known biomarkers. Treatment options are listed in Guide 8 and Guide 9 based on cancer type and performance status.

Performance status

Your performance status is your ability to do activities. It is used by doctors as a measure of general health. If your health is poor, some treatments may not be good for you. The ECOG (**E**astern **C**ooperative **O**ncology **G**roup) Performance Scale is a common scoring system. It consists of four scores.

- A **score of 0** means you are fully active.
- A **score of 1** means you are able to do all self-care activities but are unable to do hard physical work.
- A **score of 2** means you are able to do all self-care activities and spend most of waking time out of bed but are unable to do any work.
- A **score of 3** means you are unable to do all self-care activities and any work and spend most of waking time in bed.
- A **score of 4** means you are fully disabled.

Immunotherapy

Immunotherapy has become a key part of systemic treatment. Pembrolizumab with chemotherapy is standard first-line treatment. It is preferred by NCCN experts. Atezolizumab with chemotherapy is also an option for adenocarcinoma, large cell, and unknown types. Immunotherapy alone is sometimes used for next-in-line treatment.

Immunotherapy regimens may be options if you're healthy enough. Often, people with low performance scores can take it. Also, immunotherapy must be likely to work and be safe for you. Read the section, *PD-L1 ≥1%,* for more information.

What to expect: Immunotherapy

- ✓ PD-1 and PD-L1 inhibitors are slowly injected into a vein (infusion). It may take 30 or 60 minutes to get the full dose.
- ✓ Infusions are given every 2 or 3 weeks.
- ✓ Common side effects include feeling tired despite sleep. It is also common to feel constipated, nauseated, and not hungry. You may have muscle or bone pain.
- ✓ Any organ can become inflamed. This is rare but can cause severe side effects.
- ✓ Tell your doctor if you are pregnant, trying to get pregnant, or are breastfeeding. Immunotherapy may harm babies.

Guide 8. Treatment for adenocarcinoma, large cell, unknown types

First-line treatment

Performance score	What are the options?
0 or 1	• Pembrolizumab + (carboplatin or cisplatin) + pemetrexed (preferred) • Atezolizumab + carboplatin + paclitaxel + bevacizumab • Platinum-doublet chemotherapy ± bevacizumab • Other types of chemotherapy
2	• Platinum-doublet or other types of chemotherapy
3 or 4	• Supportive care

Next-in-line treatment

Performance score	What are the options?
0 or 1 or 2	• Nivolumab or pembrolizumab or atezolizumab (preferred) • Docetaxel or pemetrexed or gemcitabine or ramucirumab + docetaxel
3 or 4	• Supportive care

Guide 9. Treatment for squamous cell carcinoma

First-line treatment

Performance score	What are the options?
0 or 1	• Pembrolizumab + carboplatin + paclitaxel (preferred) • Pembrolizumab + cisplatin + paclitaxel • Platinum-doublet or other types of chemotherapy
2	• Platinum-based or other types of chemotherapy
3 or 4	• Supportive care

Next-in-line treatment

Performance score	What are the options?
0 or 1 or 2	• Nivolumab or pembrolizumab or atezolizumab (preferred) • Docetaxel or pemetrexed or ramucirumab + docetaxel
3 or 4	• Supportive care

VEGF-targeted therapy

Cancer cells need blood to grow. They send VEGF (**v**ascular **e**ndothelial **g**rowth **f**actor) to endothelial cells to start the growth of blood vessels. Unlike other biomarkers, VEGF is not mutated. However, it plays a role in most lung cancers.

VEGF-targeted therapy stops the growth of new blood vessels. **See Figure 8**. Often, people with low performance scores can have this treatment. Bevacizumab with platinum-doublet chemotherapy is used to treat adenocarcinomas, large cell, and unknown types. Ramucirumab with docetaxel may be an option for next-in-line treatment.

Figure 8
VEGF-targeted therapy

Cancer cells need blood to grow. Bevacizumab and ramucirumab stop endothelial cells from forming new blood vessels on tumors. Both are given by infusion. Ask your treatment team for a full list of side effects.

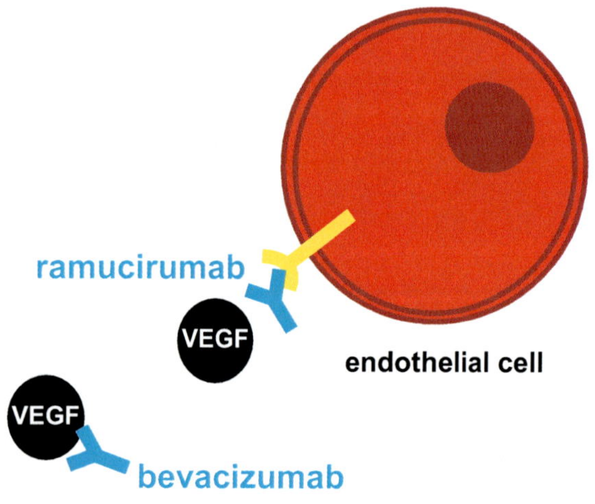

Chemotherapy

For first-line treatment, cisplatin or carboplatin—drugs made with platinum—is often used with another chemotherapy. These regimens are called platinum-doublet chemotherapy. Side effects may be severe, so you must be healthy enough to take them.

Single agents may be used if your performance score is 2. These agents include albumin-bound paclitaxel, docetaxel, gemcitabine, and paclitaxel. Pemetrexed may be an option for adenocarcinomas, large cell, and unknown types.

If there's no cancer growth, a total of 4 to 6 chemotherapy cycles are advised. Afterward, you may stay on some of your first-line treatments. This is called continuation maintenance. Another option is changing to a medicine that you didn't take as a first-line treatment. This is called switch maintenance. A third option is to start to watch and wait (observation).

Clinical trial

Joining a clinical trial may be an option for lung cancer treatment. Ask your treatment team if there is a clinical trial you can join. Also ask about the pros and cons of the trial.

Supportive care

A performance score of 3 or 4 suggests that cancer drugs will be too harmful. Therefore, the best supportive care is advised. Supportive care aims to treat the symptoms caused by the cancer.

What to expect: Chemotherapy

- ✓ Chemotherapy works by stopping the cell life cycle. As a result, cancer cells cannot make new cells. Chemotherapy can also cause cells to destroy themselves.
- ✓ It is slowly injected into a vein (infusion) but sometimes it is made as a pill.
- ✓ It is given in cycles of treatment days followed by days of rest. The cycles vary in length depending on which drugs are used.
- ✓ In general, side effects are caused by the death of fast-growing cells. Such side effects include not feeling hungry, nausea, vomiting, diarrhea, hair loss, and mouth sores.

Review

- The aim of treatment is to reduce symptoms, control the cancer, and extend life.
- Targeted therapy is used to treat lung cancer with EGFR, ALK, ROS1, BRAF V600E, and *NTRK* markers.
- Immunotherapy with or without chemotherapy is used to treat lung cancer that has PD-L1 ≥1%.
- If you are healthy enough, metastatic disease with no known markers is first treated with systemic therapy. Immunotherapy with chemotherapy is standard treatment. Bevacizumab may be added. If these combined treatments may be harmful, chemotherapy alone or supportive care may be given.

"I qualified for a clinical trial. Tumor has reduced in size by almost two-thirds and fluid cleared. Right now I'm doing great and my horizon has lengthened considerably. Grateful to be a "survivor."

– Fred
Lung cancer survivor

4 Making treatment decisions

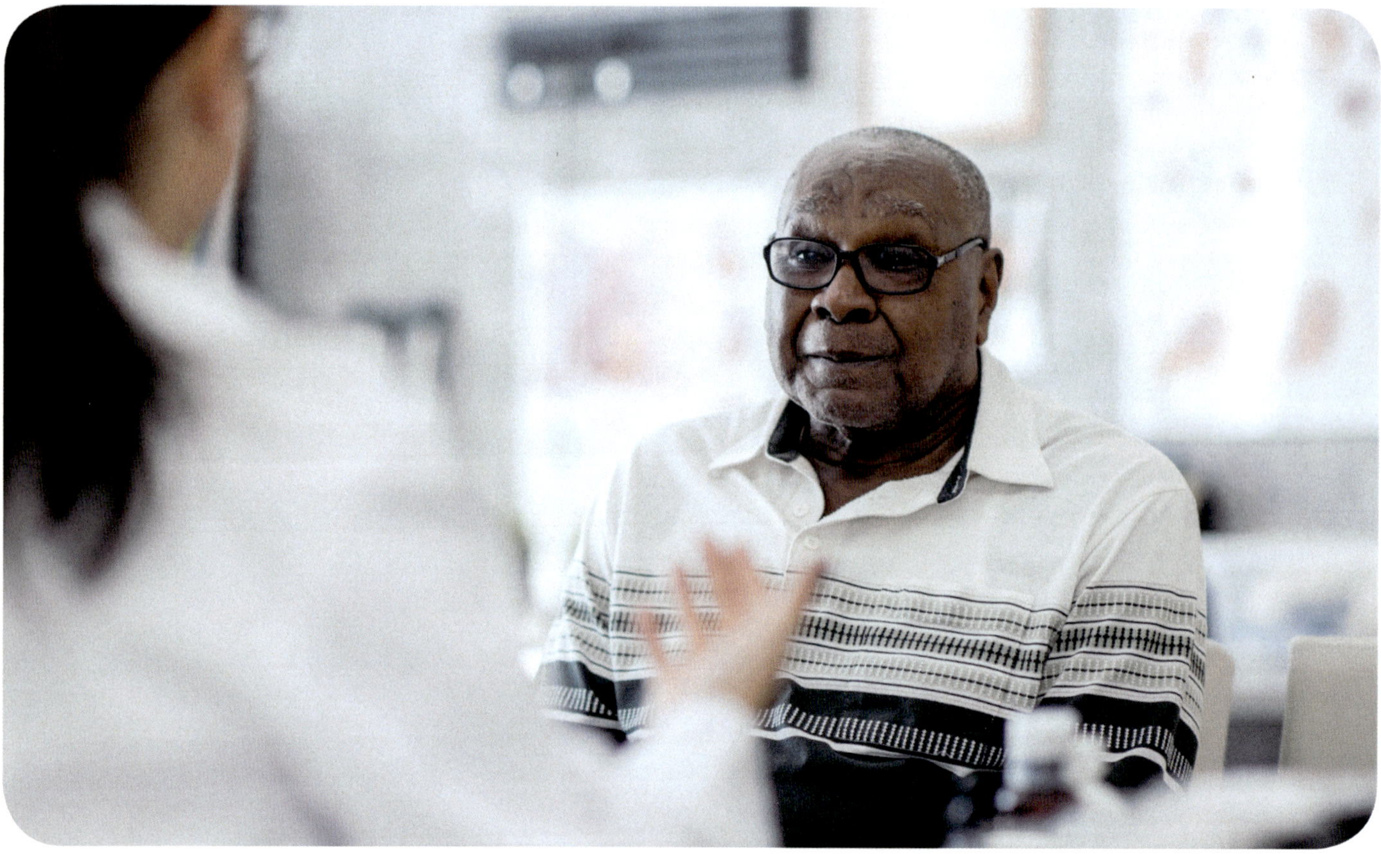

Having cancer is very stressful. While absorbing the fact that you have cancer, you have to learn about tests and treatments. In addition, the time you have to accept a treatment plan feels short. Parts 1 through 3 described the cancer and treatment options. This chapter aims to help you make decisions that are in line with your beliefs, wishes, and values.

It's your choice

The role each person wants in choosing his or her treatment differs. You may feel uneasy about making treatment decisions. This may be due to a high level of stress. It may be hard to hear or know what others are saying. Stress, pain, and drugs can limit your ability to make good decisions. You may feel uneasy because you don't know much about cancer. You've never heard the words used to describe cancer, tests, or treatments. Likewise, you may think that your judgment isn't any better than your doctors'.

Letting others decide which option is best may make you feel more at ease. But, whom do you want to make the decisions? You may rely on your doctors alone to make the right decisions. However, your doctors may not tell you which option to choose if you have multiple good options. You can also have loved ones help. They can gather information, speak on your behalf, and share in decision-making with your doctors. Even if others decide which treatment you will receive, you still have to agree by signing a consent form.

On the other hand, you may want to take the lead or share in decision-making. Most patients do. In shared decision-making, you and your doctors share information, weigh the options, and agree on a treatment plan. Your doctors know the science behind your plan but you know your concerns and goals. By working together, you are likely to get a higher quality of care and be more satisfied. You'll likely get the treatment you want, at the place you want, and by the doctors you want.

Questions to ask your doctors

You may meet with experts from different fields of medicine. Strive to have helpful talks with each person. Prepare questions before your visit and ask questions if the person isn't clear. You can also take notes and get copies of your medical records.

It may be helpful to have your spouse, partner, family member, or a friend with you at these visits. A patient advocate or navigator might also be able to come. They can help to ask questions and remember what was said. Suggested questions to ask are listed on the following pages.

"

When you are diagnosed with cancer, the most important thing that you can arm yourself with is knowledge and education.

– Anonymous
Lung cancer survivor

What's my diagnosis and prognosis?

It's important to know that there are different types of cancer. Cancer can greatly differ even when people have a tumor in the same organ. Based on your test results, your doctor can tell you which type of cancer you have. He or she can also give a prognosis. A prognosis is the likely course and outcome of a disease based on tests. Be aware, it is based on what your doctor has seen in patients like you. Knowing the prognosis may affect what you decide about treatment.

1. Where did the cancer start? In what type of cell? Is this cancer common?
2. What is the cancer stage? Does this stage mean the cancer has spread far?
3. What tests do you recommend for me?
4. Where will the tests take place? How long will the tests take and will any test hurt?
5. What if I am pregnant?
6. How do I prepare for testing?
7. Should I bring a list of my medications?
8. Should I bring someone with me?
9. How often are these tests wrong?
10. Will the biopsy remove a large enough sample for biomarker (molecular) testing?
11. Would you give me a copy of the pathology report and other test results?
12. Who will talk with me about the next steps? When?

What are my options?

There is no single treatment practice that is best for all people. There is often more than one treatment option along with clinical trial options. Your doctor will review your test results and recommend treatment options.

1. What will happen if I do nothing?
2. Can I just carefully monitor the cancer?
3. Do you consult NCCN recommendations when considering options?
4. Are you suggesting options other than what NCCN recommends? If yes, why?
5. Do your suggested options include clinical trials? Please explain why.
6. How do my age, health, and other factors affect my options? What if I am pregnant?
7. Which option is proven to work best?
8. Which options lack scientific proof?
9. What are the benefits of each option? Does any option offer a cure or long-term cancer control? Are my chances any better for one option than another? Less time-consuming? Less expensive?
10. What are the risks of each option? What are possible complications? What are the rare and common side effects? Short-lived and long-lasting side effects? Serious or mild side effects? Other risks?
11. How do you know if treatment is working?
12. What are my options if treatment doesn't working?
13. What can be done to prevent or relieve the side effects of treatment?

What does each option require of me?

Many patients consider how each option will practically affect their lives. This information may be important because you have family, jobs, and other duties to take care of. You also may be concerned about getting the help you need. If you have more than one option, choosing the option that is the least taxing may be important to you.

1. Will I have to go to the hospital or elsewhere? How often? How long is each visit?
2. What do I need to think about if I will travel for treatment?
3. Do I have a choice of when to begin treatment? Can I choose the days and times of treatment?
4. How do I prepare for treatment? Do I have to stop taking any of my medicines? Are there foods I will have to avoid?
5. Should I bring someone with me when I get treated?
6. Will the treatment hurt?
7. How much will the treatment cost me? What does my insurance cover?
8. Will I miss work or school? Will I be able to drive?
9. Is home care after treatment needed? If yes, what type?
10. How soon will I be able to manage my own health?
11. When will I be able to return to my normal activities?

What is your experience?

More and more research is finding that patients treated by more experienced doctors have better results. It is important to learn if a doctor is an expert in the cancer treatment he or she is offering.

1. Are you board-certified? If yes, in what area?
2. How many patients like me have you treated?
3. How many procedures like the one you're suggesting have you done?
4. Is this treatment a major part of your practice?
5. How many of your patients have had complications?

Deciding between options

Deciding which option is best can be hard. Doctors from different fields of medicine may have different opinions on which option is best for you. This can be very confusing. Your spouse or partner may disagree with which option you want. This can be stressful. In some cases, one option hasn't been shown to work better than another. Some ways to decide on treatment are discussed next.

2nd opinion

The time around deciding a treatment is very stressful. People with cancer often want to get treated as soon as possible. They want to make their cancer go away before it spreads farther. While cancer can't be ignored, usually there is time to think about and choose which option is best for you.

You may wish to have another doctor review your test results and suggest a treatment plan. This is called getting a 2nd opinion. You may completely trust your doctor, but a 2nd opinion about which option is best can help.

Copies of the pathology report, imaging, and other test results need to be sent to the doctor giving the 2nd opinion. Some people feel uneasy asking for copies from their doctors. However, a 2nd opinion is a normal part of cancer care.

When doctors have cancer, most will talk with more than one doctor before choosing their treatment. What's more, some health plans require a 2nd opinion. If your health plan doesn't cover the cost of a 2nd opinion, you have the choice of paying for it yourself.

If the two opinions are the same, you may feel more at peace about the treatment you accept to have. If the two opinions differ, think about getting a 3rd opinion. A 3rd opinion may help you decide between your options. Choosing your cancer treatment is a very important decision. It can affect your length and quality of life.

Support groups

Besides talking to health experts, it may help to talk to other people who have walked in your shoes. At support groups, you can ask questions and hear about the experiences of other people with lung cancer. Find a support group at the websites listed in the next section.

Compare benefits and downsides

Every option has benefits and downsides. Consider these when deciding which option is best for you. Talking to others can help identify benefits and downsides you haven't thought of. Scoring each factor from 0 to 10 can also help since some factors may be more important to you than others.

Websites

American Cancer Society
cancer.org/cancer/lung-cancer.html

American Lung Association
lung.org

Bonnie J. Addario Lung Cancer Foundation
lungcancerfoundation.org

Caring Ambassadors Program, Inc.
lungcancercap.org

Dusty Joy Foundation (LiveLung)
LiveLung.org

Free ME from Lung Cancer
freeMEfromLungCancer.org

Lung Cancer Action Network (LungCan)
LungCAN.org

Lung Cancer Alliance
lungcanceralliance.org

Lung Cancer Circle of Hope
lungcancercircleofhope.org

Lung Cancer Initiative of North Carolina
lungcancerinitiativenc.org

Lung Cancer Research Foundation
lcrf.org

LUNGevity Foundation
LUNGevity.org

National Cancer Institute (NCI)
cancer.gov/types/lung

National Coalition for Cancer Survivorship
canceradvocacy.org/toolbox

NCCN for Patients®
nccn.org/patients

Help Services

American Lung Association
Join the Better Breathers Club to learn ways to cope with lung disease.

Bonnie J. Addario Lung Cancer Foundation
Join the monthly Lung Cancer Living Room to get key information and support.

Caring Ambassadors
Order free educational materials on lung cancer.

Dusty Joy foundation (LiveLung)
Join online or in-person support groups.

Free ME from Lung Cancer
Learn basics About Lung Cancer.

Lung Cancer Action Network (LungCAN)
Learn about many patient services at Access Patient Services.

Lung Cancer Alliance
Call 1-800-298-2436 or email support@lungcanceralliance.org for help with treatment.

Lung Cancer Initiative of North Carolina
Meet fellow survivors through a local Survivor's Meet & Mingle.

Lung Cancer Research Foundation
Get matched to clinical trials in 60 seconds with Antidote.

LUNGevity Foundation
Receive one-on-one support through the LifeLine Support Partners program.

Review

- Shared decision-making is a process in which you and your doctors plan treatment together.
- Asking your doctors questions is vital to getting the information you need to make informed decisions.
- Getting a 2nd opinion, attending support groups, and comparing benefits and downsides may help you decide which treatment is best for you.

Words to know

adenocarcinoma
A cancer of cells that line organs and make fluids or hormones.

adrenal gland
A small organ on top of each kidney that makes hormones.

AJCC
American Joint Committee on Cancer

ALK
anaplastic lymphoma kinase

alveoli
The tiny sacs in the lungs where gases are transferred in and out of the blood.

anaplastic lymphoma kinase (ALK)
A type of protein on the edge of a cell that sends signals for cell growth.

biomarker
Any molecule in your body that can be measured to assess your health.

biomarker testing
Tests of any molecule in your body that can be measured to assess your health. Also called molecular testing.

biopsy
A procedure that removes fluid or tissue samples to be tested for a disease.

board certified
A status for doctors who finished training in a specialized field of medicine.

body plethysmograph
A test of how much air is in your lungs after inhaling or exhaling.

bronchi
The two airways extending from the windpipe into the lungs.

bronchioli
Small airways within the lungs.

bronchus
One of the two main airways that extends into the lungs.

cancer stage
A rating of the outlook of a cancer based on its growth and spread.

carcinoma
A cancer of cells that line the inner or outer surfaces of the body.

CBC
complete blood count

chemoradiation
A cancer treatment with both cell-killing drugs and high-energy rays.

chemistry profile
A lab test of the amount of 8 chemicals in a sample of blood. Also called metabolic panel.

chemotherapy
Cancer drugs that stop the cell life cycle so cells don't increase in number.

clinical stage
The rating of the extent of cancer before treatment is started.

clinical trial
A type of research that assesses how well health tests or treatments work in people.

complete blood count (CBC)
A lab test that measures the parts of the blood.

computed tomography (CT)
A test that uses x-rays from many angles to make a picture of the insides of the body.

continuation maintenance
A treatment phase using one or more first-line drugs to prolong good treatment results.

contrast
A dye put into your body to make clearer pictures during imaging.

core needle biopsy
A procedure that removes tissue samples with a hollow needle. Also called core biopsy.

CT
computed tomography

diagnosis
An identification of an illness based on tests.

DNA
deoxyribonucleic acid

doublet chemotherapy
A treatment with two drugs that kill cancer cells.

EBUS
endobronchial ultrasound

EBUS-TBNA
endobronchial ultrasound-guided transbronchial needle aspiration

ECOG
Eastern Cooperative Oncology Group

EGFR
epidermal growth factor receptor

endoscopic ultrasound–guided fine needle aspiration (EUS-FNA)
A procedure that removes fluid with a needle on an imaging device guided through a natural opening.

endobronchial ultrasound–guided transbronchial needle aspiration (EBUS-TBNA)
A procedure that removes lung tissue with a needle on an imaging device guided down the windpipe.

epidermal growth factor receptor (EGFR)
A protein on the edge of a cell that sends signals to the cell to grow.

EUS
endoscopic ultrasound

EUS-FNA
endoscopic ultrasound-guided fine-needle aspiration

FDG
fluorodeoxyglucose

fine-needle aspiration (FNA)
A procedure that removes tissue samples with a very thin needle.

FNA
fine-needle aspiration

gas diffusion
A test that uses harmless gas to measure how much you can breathe out.

gene
Coded instructions in cells for making new cells and controlling how cells behave.

gene rearrangement
A coded instruction within a cell that is made from parts of other coded instructions.

HER2
human epidermal growth factor receptor 2

human epidermal growth factor receptor 2 (HER2)
A protein on the edge of a cell that sends signals to the cell to grow.

immunotherapy
A treatment with drugs that help the body find and destroy cancer cells.

invasion
The growth of cancer cells from where it started into another tissue.

large-cell lung carcinoma
A cancer of lung cells that lack features to classify as another type of lung cancer.

lobe
A clearly seen division in an organ.

lymph
A clear fluid containing white blood cells.

lymph node
A small, bean-shaped, disease-fighting structure.

magnetic resonance imaging (MRI)
A test that uses radio waves and powerful magnets to make pictures of the insides of the body.

maintenance treatment
A treatment phase that is given to prolong good treatment results.

medical history
A report of all your health events and medications.

metastasis
he spread of cancer from the first tumor to a new site.

MRI
magnetic resonance imaging

molecular testing
A lab test of any molecule in your body that can be measured to assess your health. Also called biomarker testing.

mutation
Abnormal changes in coded instructions within cells (genes).

NCCN
National Comprehensive Cancer Network

non-small cell lung cancer (NSCLC)
A cancer that starts in lung cells that are not small.

NSCLC
non-small cell lung cancer

observation
A period of testing for changes in cancer status while not receiving treatment.

parietal pleura
The outer layer of the tissue lining around the lungs.

pathologic stage
A rating of the extent of cancer based on tests given after treatment.

pathologist
A doctor who's an expert in testing cells and tissue to find disease.

performance status
A rating of one's ability to do daily activities.

pericardiocentesis
A procedure that removes fluid from around the heart with a needle.

PET
positron emission tomography

physical exam
A review of the body by a health expert for signs of disease.

platinum-doublet chemotherapy
A treatment with two cell-killing drugs, one of which contains the chemical platinum.

pleura
The two layers of tissue lining around the lungs.

pleural cavity
The space between the two layers of tissue lining around the lungs.

pleural effusion
An excess of fluid between the two layers of tissue lining around the lungs.

pleural fluid
The liquid in the space between the two layers of the tissue lining the lungs.

positron emission tomography (PET)
A test that uses radioactive material to see the shape and function of body parts.

positron emission tomography/computed tomography (PET/CT)
A test that uses two picture-making methods to show the shape and function of tissue.

primary tumor
The first mass of a certain type of cancer cells.

prognosis
The likely course and outcome of a disease based on tests.

pulmonary function tests
A set of breathing tests to test the strength of the lungs.

radiation oncologist
A doctor who's an expert in treating cancer with radiation.

radiation therapy
A treatment that uses intense energy to kill cancer cells.

respiratory system
The group of organs that transfers gases in and out of the body.

ROS1
A type of protein on the edge of a cell that sends signals for cell growth.

secondary tumor
A mass of cancer cells that formed from the first mass of cancer cells.

side effect
An unhealthy or unpleasant physical or emotional response to treatment.

small cell lung cancer
A cancer of small, round lung cells.

spirometry
A test that uses a tube to measure how fast you breathe.

squamous cell carcinoma
A type of cancer of thin and flat cells that line the surface of organs.

supportive care
Health care that includes symptom relief but not cancer treatment. Also sometimes called palliative care.

surgery
An operation to remove or repair a part of the body.

switch maintenance
A treatment phase with a new drug that is given to prolong good treatment results.

targeted therapy
A drug treatment that impedes the growth process specific to cancer cells.

thoracic radiologist
A doctor who's an expert in reading imaging tests of the chest.

thoracoscopy
A procedure to do work in the chest with a device passed through a small cut in the skin. Also called VATS.

trachea
The airway between the throat and airway into the lungs. Also called the windpipe.

transthoracic needle aspiration (TTNA)
A procedure that removes tissue samples with a thin needle guided through the ribs.

TTNA
transthoracic needle aspiration

ultrasound
A test that uses sound waves to take pictures of the inside of the body.

vascular endothelial growth factor (VEGF)
A molecule that triggers the growth of blood vessels.

VEGF
vascular endothelial growth factor

visceral pleura
The inner layer of tissue lining around the lungs.

NCCN Contributors

This patient guide is based on the NCCN Clinical Practice Guidelines in Oncology (NCCN Guidelines®) for Non-Small Cell Lung Cancer. It was adapted, reviewed, and published with help from the following people:

Dorothy A. Shead, MS
Director, Patient Information Operations

Laura J. Hanisch, PsyD
Medical Writer/Patient Information Specialist

Erin Vidic, MA
Medical Writer

Tanya Fischer, MEd, MSLIS
Medical Writer

Rachael Clarke
Senior Medical Copyeditor

Kim Williams
Creative Services Manager

Susan Kidney
Design Specialist

The NCCN Clinical Practice Guidelines in Oncology (NCCN Guidelines®) for Non-Small Cell Lung Cancer, Version 5.2019 were developed by the following NCCN Panel Members:

David S. Ettinger, MD/Chair
The Sidney Kimmel Comprehensive Cancer Center at Johns Hopkins

Douglas E. Wood, MD/Vice Chair
Fred Hutchinson Cancer Research Center/Seattle Cancer Care Alliance

Charu Aggarwal, MD, MPH
Abramson Cancer Center at the University of Pennsylvania

Dara L. Aisner, MD, PhD
University of Colorado Cancer Center

Wallace Akerley, MD
Huntsman Cancer Institute at the University of Utah

Jessica Bauman, MD
Fox Chase Cancer Center

Ankit Bharat, MD
Robert H. Lurie Comprehensive Cancer Center of Northwestern University

Debora Bruno, MD
Case Comprehensive Cancer Center/ University Hospitals Seidman Cancer Center and Cleveland Clinic Taussig Cancer Institute

Joe Y. Chang, MD, PhD
The University of Texas MD Anderson Cancer Center

Lucian R. Chirieac, MD
Dana-Farber/Brigham and Women's Cancer Center

Thomas A. D'Amico, MD
Duke Cancer Institute

Thomas J. Dilling, MD, MS
Moffitt Cancer Center

Michael Dobelbower, MD, PhD
O'Neal Comprehensive Cancer Center at UAB

Ramaswamy Govindan, MD
Siteman Cancer Center at Barnes-Jewish Hospital and Washington University School of Medicine

Matthew A. Gubens, MD, MS
UCSF Helen Diller Family Comprehensive Cancer Center

Mark Hennon, MD
Roswell Park Cancer Institute

Leora Horn, MD, MSc
Vanderbilt-Ingram Cancer Center

Rudy P. Lackner, MD
Fred & Pamela Buffett Cancer Center

Michael Lanuti, MD
Massachusetts General Hospital Cancer Center

Ticiana A. Leal, MD
University of Wisconsin Carbone Cancer Center

Rogerio Lilenbaum, MD
Yale Cancer Center/ Smilow Cancer Hospital

Jules Lin, MD
University of Michigan Rogel Cancer Center

Billy W. Loo, Jr., MD, PhD
Stanford Cancer Institute

Renato Martins, MD, MPH
Fred Hutchinson Cancer Research Center/ Seattle Cancer Care Alliance

*Gregory A. Otterson, MD
The Ohio State University Comprehensive Cancer Center - James Cancer Hospital and Solove Research Institute

Sandip P. Patel, MD
UC San Diego Moores Cancer Center

Karen Reckamp, MD, MS
City of Hope National Medical Center

Gregory J. Riely, MD, PhD
Memorial Sloan Kettering Cancer Center

Steven E. Schild, MD
Mayo Clinic Cancer Center

Theresa A. Shapiro, MD, PhD
The Sidney Kimmel Comprehensive Cancer Center at Johns Hopkins

James Stevenson, MD
Case Comprehensive Cancer Center/ University Hospitals Seidman Cancer Center and Cleveland Clinic Taussig Cancer Institute

Scott J. Swanson, MD
Dana-Farber/Brigham and Women's Cancer Center

Kurt Tauer, MD
St. Jude Children's Research Hospital/ University of Tennessee Health Science Center

Stephen C. Yang, MD
The Sidney Kimmel Comprehensive Cancer Center at Johns Hopkins

NCCN Staff

Kristina M. Gregory, RN, MSN, OCN
Vice President/Clinical Information Operations

Miranda Hughes, PhD
Oncology Scientist/Senior Medical Writer

* Reviewed this patient guide.
For disclosures, visit www.nccn.org/about/disclosure.aspx.

NCCN Cancer Centers

Abramson Cancer Center
at the University of Pennsylvania
Philadelphia, Pennsylvania
800.789.7366
pennmedicine.org/cancer

Fred & Pamela Buffett Cancer Center
Omaha, Nebraska
800.999.5465
nebraskamed.com/cancer

Case Comprehensive Cancer Center/
University Hospitals Seidman Cancer
Center and Cleveland Clinic Taussig
Cancer Institute
Cleveland, Ohio
800.641.2422 • UH Seidman Cancer Center
uhhospitals.org/seidman
866.223.8100 • CC Taussig Cancer Institute
my.clevelandclinic.org/services/cancer
216.844.8797 • Case CCC
case.edu/cancer

City of Hope National Medical Center
Los Angeles, California
800.826.4673
cityofhope.org

Dana-Farber/Brigham and
Women's Cancer Center
Massachusetts General Hospital
Cancer Center
Boston, Massachusetts
877.332.4294
dfbwcc.org
massgeneral.org/cancer

Duke Cancer Institute
Durham, North Carolina
888.275.3853
dukecancerinstitute.org

Fox Chase Cancer Center
Philadelphia, Pennsylvania
888.369.2427
foxchase.org

Huntsman Cancer Institute
at the University of Utah
Salt Lake City, Utah
877.585.0303
huntsmancancer.org

Fred Hutchinson Cancer
Research Center/Seattle
Cancer Care Alliance
Seattle, Washington
206.288.7222 • seattlecca.org
206.667.5000 • fredhutch.org

The Sidney Kimmel Comprehensive
Cancer Center at Johns Hopkins
Baltimore, Maryland
410.955.8964
hopkinskimmelcancercenter.org

Robert H. Lurie Comprehensive
Cancer Center of Northwestern
University
Chicago, Illinois
866.587.4322
cancer.northwestern.edu

Mayo Clinic Cancer Center
Phoenix/Scottsdale, Arizona
Jacksonville, Florida
Rochester, Minnesota
800.446.2279 • Arizona
904.953.0853 • Florida
507.538.3270 • Minnesota
www.mayoclinic.org/cancercenter

Memorial Sloan Kettering
Cancer Center
New York, New York
800.525.2225
mskcc.org

Moffitt Cancer Center
Tampa, Florida
800.456.3434
moffitt.org

The Ohio State University
Comprehensive Cancer Center -
James Cancer Hospital and
Solove Research Institute
Columbus, Ohio
800.293.5066
cancer.osu.edu

O'Neal Comprehensive
Cancer Center at UAB
Birmingham, Alabama
800.822.0933
uab.edu/onealcancercenter/

Roswell Park Comprehensive
Cancer Center
Buffalo, New York
877.275.7724
roswellpark.org

Siteman Cancer Center at Barnes-
Jewish Hospital and Washington
University School of Medicine
St. Louis, Missouri
800.600.3606
siteman.wustl.edu

St. Jude Children's
Research Hospital
The University of Tennessee
Health Science Center
Memphis, Tennessee
888.226.4343 • stjude.org
901.683.0055 • westclinic.com

Stanford Cancer Institute
Stanford, California
877.668.7535
cancer.stanford.edu

UC San Diego Moores Cancer Center
La Jolla, California
858.657.7000
cancer.ucsd.edu

UCSF Helen Diller Family
Comprehensive Cancer Center
San Francisco, California
800.689.8273
cancer.ucsf.edu

University of Colorado Cancer Center
Aurora, Colorado
720.848.0300
coloradocancercenter.org

University of Michigan
Rogel Cancer Center
Ann Arbor, Michigan
800.865.1125
mcancer.org

The University of Texas
MD Anderson Cancer Center
Houston, Texas
800.392.1611
mdanderson.org

University of Wisconsin
Carbone Cancer Center
Madison, Wisconsin
608.265.1700
uwhealth.org/cancer

Vanderbilt-Ingram Cancer Center
Nashville, Tennessee
800.811.8480
vicc.org

Yale Cancer Center/
Smilow Cancer Hospital
New Haven, Connecticut
855.4.SMILOW
yalecancercenter.org

Index

Made in the USA
Las Vegas, NV
26 March 2021

20211216R00033